# PRAISE FOR *THE PALEOVEDIC DIET*

"Integrative medicine expert Dr. Akil Palanisamy makes both timeless knowledge and leading-edge research accessible in this groundbreaking and timely book. *The Paleovedic Diet* is rich with useful information on such diverse issues as gluten sensitivity, the human microbiome, detoxification in modern times and the rise of autoimmune disease. *The Paleovedic Diet* is a must-read for anyone serious about achieving optimal health and vitality."
—Andrew Weil, MD, world-renowned integrative medicine physician and bestselling author

"The Paleovedic Diet represents the best of integrative medicine, combining ancient wisdom with modern science and functional medicine to create a definitive roadmap to health. In an engaging and easy to read style, Dr. Akil presents the most up-to-date, evidence-based health information available today. He sheds light on topics such as optimal nutrition, the 100 trillion bacteria that make up your microbiome, the best way to exercise, and powerful detox practices. He reveals the hidden healing powers of spices and shows you how to use Ayurveda to customize a diet that's best for you. *The Paleovedic Diet* can help you lose weight, increase energy, and reverse disease."
—Mark Hyman, MD, eight-time #1 *New York Times*–bestselling author and functional medicine expert

"Dr. Akil deftly weaves the ancient wisdom of Ayurveda together with the principles of a nutrient-dense, Paleolithic diet to create a practical, individualized approach to wellness. If you've been looking for a way of eating and living that is tailored especially for your body and mind, this book is for you."
—Chris Kresser, LAc, *New York Times*–bestselling author of *The Paleo Cure*

"An impressively powerful intersection between East, West, and Ancestral Health. *The Paleovedic Diet* gives you a comprehensive guide to optimal health that integrates time-tested recommendations from ancient cultures along with the hard modern science that backs up their efficacy. Every page is chock full of invaluable, evidence-based guidelines on how to individualize your health plan for success. It's a truly impressive collection of information."
—Mark Sisson, *New York Times*–bestselling author of *The Primal Blueprint*

"In *The Paleovedic Diet*, Dr. Akil integrates his extensive clinical experience, the latest scientific research, and the most effective aspects of the Paleo diet with Ayurveda, the time-tested traditional medical system of India. He has created an enlightening, customizable, and easily actionable roadmap to optimal health that will open your eyes. *The Paleovedic Diet* has changed my approach to healthy living—and it'll change yours, too." —Michelle Tam, *New York Times*–bestselling author of *Nom Nom Paleo: Food For Humans*

"*The Paleovedic Diet* is a powerful synthesis of the healing wisdom of a thousand years of ancient medicine and the precision and clear thinking of the best of scientific method. In elegant and easily accessible language, Dr. Akil Palanisamy makes available to us a wealth of previously unknown information about ourselves and the resolution of our most common problems. It is impossible to read this book without finding something in it that will heal you. A brilliant contribution to the health of every one of us." —Rachel Naomi Remen, MD, *New York Times*–bestselling author of *Kitchen Table Wisdom* and *My Grandfather's Blessings*

"If you have been increasingly confused about what to eat, this is the book for you! Dr. Akil provides a sage and easy to follow middle way that blends the best of medical science with the wisdom of ancestral traditions." —Victoria Maizes, MD, Executive Director, Arizona Center for Integrative Medicine

"Dr. Akil has beautifully blended the ancient, timeless wisdom of Ayurveda and Ayurvedic principles of healing with the light of modern medicine, integrated so that anyone can use it for his or her total healing." —Vasant Lad, BAMS, internationally recognized Ayurvedic physician, author of *Ayurveda: Science of Self-Healing*

# THE PALEOVEDIC DIET

## A Complete Program to Burn Fat, Increase Energy, and Reverse Disease

Akil Palanisamy, MD

Foreword by Robb Wolf

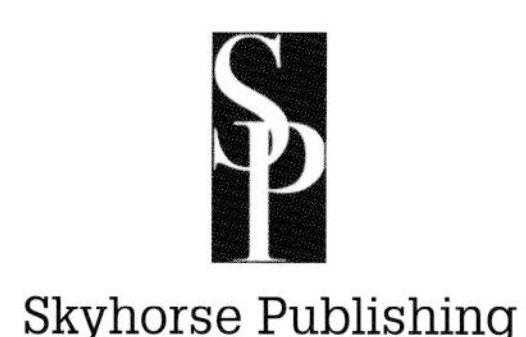

Skyhorse Publishing

First Skyhorse Publishing paperback edition, 2021.



Skyhorse Publishing books may be purchased in bulk at special discounts for sales promotion, corporate gifts, fund-raising, or educational purposes. Special editions can also be created to specifications. For details, contact the Special Sales Department, Skyhorse Publishing, 307 West 36th Street, 11th Floor, New York, NY 10018 or info@skyhorsepublishing.com.



Visit our website at www.skyhorsepublishing.com.

10 9 8 7 6 5 4 3 2 1

Library of Congress Cataloging-in-Publication Data is available on file.

Cover design by Laura Klynstra

Print ISBN: 978-1-5107-6311-1
Ebook ISBN: 978-1-5107-0067-3

Printed in China

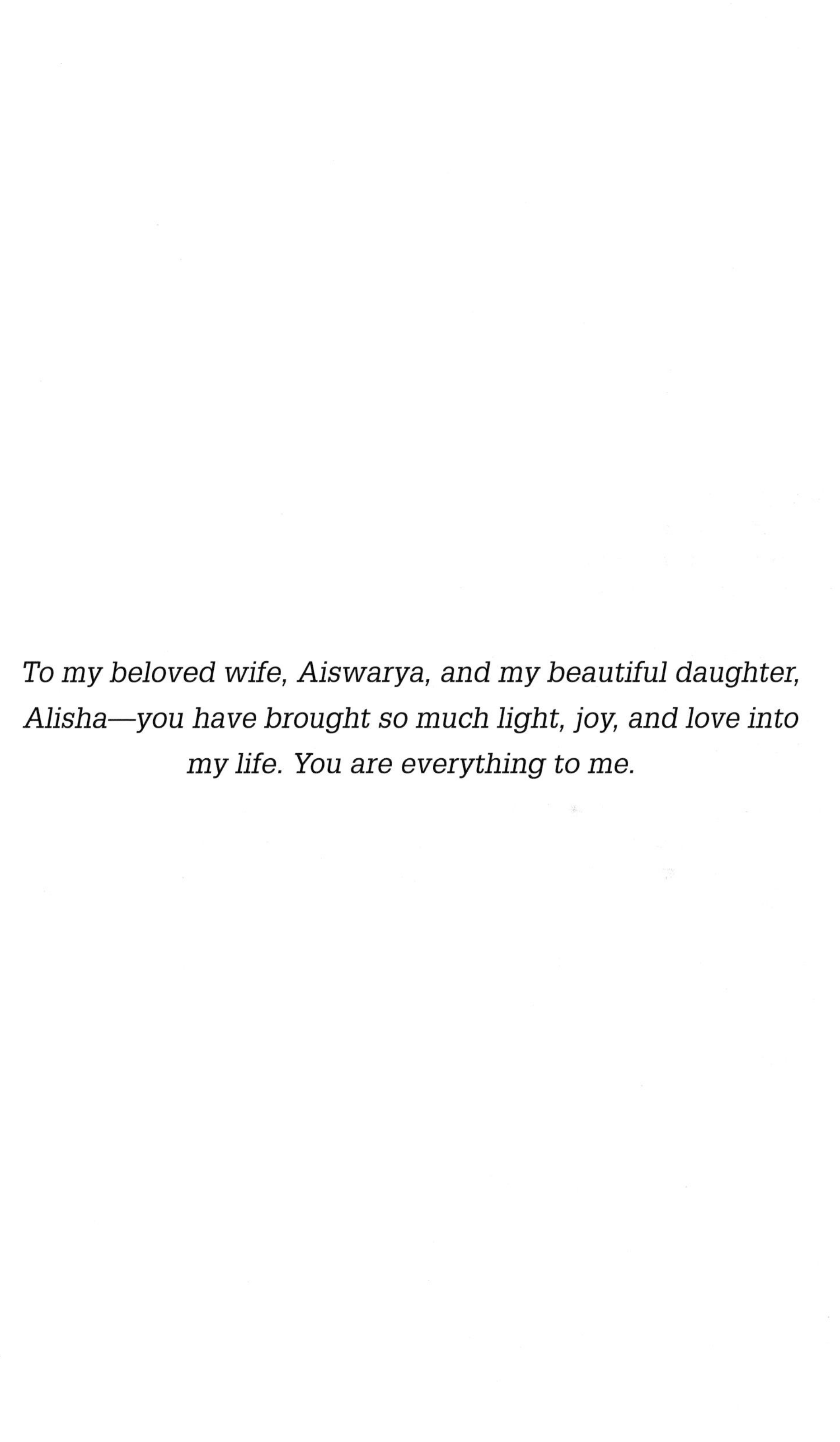

*To my beloved wife, Aiswarya, and my beautiful daughter, Alisha—you have brought so much light, joy, and love into my life. You are everything to me.*

# TABLE OF CONTENTS

## PART THREE—*Detoxify to Reach the Next Level of Health*

# DISCLAIMER

This book is intended to provide information for educational purposes only and is not intended to diagnose or treat any medical condition or illness. It is not a substitute for diagnosis and treatment prescribed by a health-care professional. If you suspect that you have a medical problem, consult a licensed health-care provider to diagnose and treat your condition. Any use of vitamins, herbs, or any nutritional supplements should be under the supervision of a trained practitioner. The author and publisher specifically disclaim any liability or loss, personal or otherwise, incurred as a consequence of the application of any of the contents of this book. Mention of specific companies or organizations in this book does not imply endorsement by the author or publisher.

# FOREWORD

"What's right for me?" It's a question I hear all the time. Personalizing the vast health information out there to find out what's best for you has been a challenge until now. *The Paleovedic Diet* provides the solution. Dr. Akil Palanisamy has integrated the latest medical research with powerful ancient wisdom to help you create a customized diet and lifestyle plan.

*The Paleovedic Diet* contains much of interest to a broad spectrum of people, ranging from Paleo aficionados to serious biohackers to innocent newbies—indeed to anyone who is really serious about optimizing his or her health. This book can help you to lose weight, boost your energy and vitality, and begin to reverse any health challenges you might be facing. "Dr. Akil" does the heavy lifting for you by reviewing and summarizing the scientific literature. There is no other physician in the world more qualified than Dr. Akil to give you accurate and reliable health information, based on his extensive experience treating thousands of complex patients.

This captivating book will take you on a whirlwind journey through a wide range of fascinating topics. In Part One, The Paleovedic Diet spotlights health-promoting secrets of long-lived societies and traditional cultures. Dr. Akil addresses every major question you might have about nutrition and dispels myths about grains and gluten, protein, good and bad fats, and exactly which fruits and vegetables to eat. He reviews the latest research about the microbiome and tells you how to optimize this vitally important but neglected human organ. He includes an impressive evidence-based review of spices, which are an incredible source of nutrients, phytochemicals, and other healing compounds that those in the Paleo world should take advantage of.

Part Two of the book covers all other important aspects of health besides nutrition. Ayurveda, which could seem esoteric, is explained in clear and practical terms to help you to understand your biochemical individuality and develop a personalized diet and lifestyle program that's right for you. Dr. Akil also discusses the importance of a daily routine, intermittent fasting, physical activity, optimal sleep, stress reduction, and balance of your mind-body connection.

In Part Three, Dr. Akil addresses a topic that is often overlooked in the Paleo realm: detoxification. He reviews startling research about the role of environmental toxins and strategies for reducing these toxins. He has created a powerful three-week detoxification protocol called The Paleovedic Detox, which can jumpstart your digestion, improve your elimination of toxins and pollutants, and help you heal from illness.

You don't have to settle for feeling bad, just getting by, or blaming your issues on getting old. You don't have to settle for anything less than perfect health. The Paleovedic Diet empowers you with the information and tools to take charge of your health and thrive. This user-friendly program has the potential to change many lives for the better, especially yours. The invitation is open—start feeling better today!

—Robb Wolf, *New York Times*–bestselling author of *The Paleo Solution*

# INTRODUCTION

## A Sobering Reality

We're in a crisis of health. Two-thirds of Americans are overweight or obese, despite spending over $50 billion a year on diet and weight-loss products. More than 100 million Americans suffer from various problems with blood sugar, ranging from mild insulin resistance to prediabetes to full-blown type 2 diabetes; by 2020, this will affect half of all Americans.[1] Fifty million Americans now suffer from allergies of some type.[2] Food allergies are especially troubling, affecting up to 10 percent of the population in some countries; rates are soaring worldwide as demonstrated by studies in the United States, United Kingdom, China, and Australia.[3]

Autoimmune disease, perhaps the most rapidly growing type of chronic disease, was virtually unknown a century ago and yet already afflicts one in ten Americans.[4] Celiac disease, an autoimmune disease characterized by gluten sensitivity, has increased in prevalence by 500 percent in the past fifty years.[5] Autoimmune type 1 diabetes has also increased by 500 percent since 1950 in certain countries, such as Finland.[6]

At the same time, we spend more as a country on health care than we've ever spent before. The amount we spend per person per year on health care, over $8,200, is the highest of any country in the world, and nearly three times more than the country that ranks second.[7] We spend around $3 trillion on health care in the United States, which is over 17 percent of GDP, the highest percentage of any country (and rising).

To be fair, the United States is a world leader in medical research and has excellent survival rates in certain diseases, like cancer. However, we still suffer from the highest obesity rates in the world, high chronic disease rates, and below-average life expectancy compared to other industrialized nations. The United States ranks forty-sixth when it comes to infant mortality, coming in behind Europe, Australia, Canada, South Korea, and Cuba.[8]

Even those of us who don't suffer from a diagnosable disease may not feel well. For example, fatigue is a widespread complaint in the United States, reported by 38 percent of people in the US workforce.[9] Nonspecific symptoms like poor digestion, brain fog, and headaches are written off as simply a result of "getting old." All of us have the basic goal of wanting to feel good and to thrive. But I meet many people who have simply given up on this goal. Many patients have come to accept low energy as a fact of life. However, after working with me for some time, they often report spectacular gains in energy and vitality.

## A Return to Basics

So what's the solution? Certainly there are social, political, and financial factors that complicate these issues. While the problem is complex, the solutions in my mind are relatively simple. They involve a return to the basics of human health, updated for the unique challenges of modern society. That's what I'm presenting in this book, based on my clinical work with thousands of patients.

It's difficult to be healthy in today's world because of environmental factors, chronic stress, isolation and lack of community, the ready availability of processed foods, and changes in our food supply. It's hard because of the explosion of conflicting, contradictory health information that inundates us from many sources. But the elements of health are present in our communities and our lives if we know what to look for and what to focus on. If we realize the importance of getting local organic food from the farmers' market, eating a diet that is right for our body type, strengthening our mind-body connection, and moving throughout the day, we could focus more on these factors.

In addition, the body has a remarkable capacity for self-healing if given the right inputs. I see many patients who have been told by other doctors that they cannot get better; however, by working with me they are often able to heal themselves.

## Myths and Misconceptions

The problem of conflicting advice and misinformation is especially acute in the realm of ancestral diet approaches that, broadly speaking, seek to emulate the dietary patterns of our ancestors. Every day I get questions from my patients about these approaches to eating. And it's clear that it is not just my patients who are interested. The Paleo Diet in particular was the most searched diet on Google worldwide in 2013—it was featured on *The Dr. Oz Show* and has become the diet of choice for people who participate in the massively popular Crossfit program.

But the level of interest in these diets is matched only by the number of myths and misconceptions about them. And with the explosion of books and websites on Paleo, it's hard to sort through the overwhelming amount of information to discern what is true and accurate. Should you eat just bacon and burgers? Since salads didn't exist in the caveman era, should you cut out vegetables? Follow a low-carb diet? (No to all of the above, FYI). It's not surprising that so many people I talk to are very confused about this subject.

## Paleo Must Be Individualized

I see many patients in my clinic who are following a Paleo diet but actually doing themselves some harm inadvertently. This may be due to consuming fewer carbohydrates than they need, not adapting their diet to changing medical conditions or life circumstances, or following a diet that is not ideal for their body type. In my experience, most people eating Paleo don't usually know that they need to customize this diet for themselves. They are always shocked to find out that the way they have been following Paleo could actually be detrimental to their health in some way. For example, eating too much raw food or eating foods that are considered "energetically heating" may be harmful depending on your Ayurvedic body type (for cases illustrating this, see Chapter 6).

## The Paleovedic Approach

It's one thing to know that "one size fits all" doesn't work in nutrition, but figuring out the diet that is best for you is much harder. To help individualize diets for my patients, I rely on Ayurveda, the five-thousand-year-old traditional medical system from India. In this book, I integrate the core principles of Paleo with the science of Ayurveda to help you determine the optimal, individualized diet for you—the Paleovedic Diet.

As a Harvard-trained M.D., I integrate a strong scientific background in biochemistry and Western medicine with training in Ayurveda and study of ancestral societies around the globe. This unique background enables me to seamlessly blend Paleo and Ayurvedic principles with the latest research in nutrition, food science, and medicine. I provide definitive, practical health information based on cutting-edge research and clinical experience.

In my practice, I incorporate an integrative medicine modality known as functional medicine, which uses specialized lab testing to diagnose and treat imbalances in the function of different organ systems. My approach has benefited thousands of patients who have utilized this approach to improve energy, lose weight, and reverse disease. The Paleovedic Diet provides practical guidelines on how to integrate the seemingly opposed worlds of ancient wisdom and modern science to create a customized nutrition plan for optimal health.

Throughout the book, cases from actual patients I have treated are included (names and identifying details are changed). I want to illustrate how people have been able to achieve radical improvements in health by following the principles discussed in the book.

## How To Use This Book

This book is divided into three parts. We begin by focusing on the health of traditional societies. There are a few areas in the world known as "blue zones," where populations still enjoy exceptional longevity and good health, such as Loma Linda, California, and Sardinia, Italy. In addition, there are a few populations that still follow a traditional hunter-gatherer diet and lifestyle, such as the Kitava people of Papua New Guinea.

Remarkably, medical analysis has revealed that these populations are relatively free of our modern illnesses like heart disease, diabetes, and cancer. What are the common elements shared by these groups? How can we apply lessons from these groups in our everyday lives?

## Part One—Fuel Your Body Optimally

Part One covers in great detail the topic of what you should put into your body, addressing popular misconceptions about ancestral eating. A question I hear frequently in my clinic is "Should I eat meat?" Some argue vehemently in favor of vegetarianism, while others emphasize the importance of animal protein. These conflicting theories are reconciled and clarified. Determining your Ayurvedic body type (which you will do in Chapter 6) can inform this decision. To me, the Paleo diet is a plant-based diet, insofar as most of your plate should be filled with vegetables. Sometimes people don't realize this, with the popular conception of Paleo as a meat-based diet.

Part One also discusses issues such as optimizing your carb intake, grains and gluten sensitivity, which types of fats are healthiest, in-depth perspectives on protein, unheralded superfoods (you'll be surprised to see what I'm talking about here), how to heal and repair your digestive tract, and a discussion of your bacterial flora and their many roles.

I then help you further refine and tailor your diet according to your Ayurvedic body type and discuss other valuable insights from Ayurveda. I review twelve powerful healing spices that comprise a veritable pharmacy of disease-fighting power. You will learn about the remarkable healing potential of each spice and get ideas about how to use them in delicious recipes. Revered in Ayurveda as medicinal agents, spices have been shown by modern research to be loaded with nutrients and phytochemicals that can help prevent or treat more than one hundred different diseases.

## Part Two—Exercise, Sleep, and the Mind-Body-Spirit Balance

Part Two addresses the other aspects of ancestral societies besides nutrition that enable them to be remarkably healthy. Before food was readily available 24/7, our ancestors had to be well-adapted to surviving alternating periods of feast and famine. A technique known as intermittent fasting that mimics this ancestral pattern of eating has been shown to help your body burn fat, balance hormones, and lose weight. Research on certain modern hunter-gatherer populations has shown that they in fact consume their food in this way.

Learning to move the way our ancestors did is vital to health. I present five secrets of optimal exercise—including a movement approach that mimics the activity pattern of hunter-gatherers in order to dramatically improve one's fitness, and in less time than it takes to do traditional workouts.

Part Two also addresses other elements that contribute to ancestral societies' well-being. This includes common practices of traditional societies that are beneficial, such as following a health-promoting daily routine, getting quality sleep, practicing stress reduction, having a sense of purpose, and maintaining a genuine connection with other people. With each topic, the focus is on simple, practical guidelines that can be implemented immediately to improve quality of life.

## Part Three—Detoxify to Reach the Next Level of Health

Part Three focuses on a core element that is often missing in the discussion of ancestral diets—the topic of detoxification. Our ancestors did not have to deal with the level of environmental pollutants and toxins that we are exposed to today. These toxins may contribute to fatigue, frequent infections, inflammation, and a host of other maladies—and you may not even realize that you have them. Through my work with patients, I have found that doing a three-week detoxification program called the "Paleovedic Detox" can take their health to the next level. This comprehensive program of diet and supplements will help you to reduce inflammation, improve energy, and detoxify.

Next, I cover common environmental toxins that we are all exposed to and may not even know about. I review the disquieting research on these toxins and provide practical suggestions on how to reduce exposures in our foods, homes, and work spaces. Tips on specific foods and practices that support daily detoxification are included. Regular cleansing and detoxification are essential for optimal health.

Part Three concludes with a detailed dietary program that puts together all the concepts from the book. Appendices include a detailed menu, food plan, and recipes by nutritionist Sharon Meyer.

## Why I Wrote This Book

I wrote this book for several reasons. First, writing has been a long-standing passion of mine and something that gives me great pleasure. Second, my patients have repeatedly asked me to write a book to describe my unique approach, which has often helped them when nothing else has. Third, I can only see so many patients in clinic each day, and I wanted to make this potentially transformative information available to anyone seeking to take charge of his or her health.

Ultimately, my goal is to present a comprehensive road map to optimal health and detail a practical, sensible, and enlightened approach to living. If enough people take control of their own health and follow a path to optimal wellness, we can alter our trajectory as a society and begin to reverse our modern epidemics of chronic disease.

> For additional resources, recipes, tips, personalized support, and more, please visit my website at www.doctorakil.com. In different parts of the book, I refer you back to the website for specific links and more detailed resources. Online you will also find bonus content that expands on the material featured in this book.

# MY STORY—WHEN MY BODY FAILED ME

Let me not pray to be sheltered from dangers,
But to be fearless in facing them.
Let me not beg for the stilling of my pain,
But for the heart to conquer it.
Let me not look for allies in life's battlefield,
But to my own strength.
Let me not crave in anxious fear to be saved,
But hope for the patience to win my freedom.
Grant me that I may not be a coward, feeling your mercy in my success alone,
But let me find the grasp of your hand in my failure.[1]

—Rabindranath Tagore, Nobel Prize–winning poet from India

I was on top of the world. I was a senior at Harvard University and had been accepted to medical school to pursue my lifelong dream of becoming a doctor. That's when the trouble started. While working on my senior thesis, I noticed severe wrist pain with numbness and tingling in my arms. The pain got worse and began to interfere with my sleep. I could no longer type on a keyboard. I went to student health services and was diagnosed with repetitive strain injury (RSI).

I had worked hard during my college years in classes and research activities, but nothing out of the ordinary. I was used to working hard and had a lot of energy to fuel that work. The previous year, I had become vegetarian. Certainly, I was under stress but managed it with a daily meditation practice. I had a regular routine of gym workouts and yoga. The reason for my illness puzzled me.

I was prescribed anti-inflammatory medication and physical therapy, and was given extra time for writing during exams and help with typing my thesis. My symptoms abated but did not disappear. I was able to finish college and graduate with honors.

I then began medical school at the University of California, San Francisco (UCSF). My top choice, UCSF was considered the premier medical school on the West Coast, and I was excited to begin. After eight years in Boston, I was eager to escape the snow as well, although the cool climate in San Francisco surprised me. I began to understand the apocryphal quote attributed to Mark Twain, "The coldest winter I ever spent was a summer in San Francisco."

I completed my first year and was happy, although I was in class all day and studied several hours each night. My symptoms had been manageable with physical therapy but began to worsen when I started my second year. The wrist pain was intolerable at times and was accompanied by back pain that made it impossible to sit for more than fifteen minutes.

Also, a heavy and onerous fatigue began to set in, which I attributed to stress. Inexplicably, I lost thirty pounds over several months from my already lean baseline weight of 138. I could not attend lectures due to worsening back pain and fatigue. I was given extra time for exams, which helped me to pass my exams and not flunk out of medical school, but I began to struggle with severe anxiety, which had never bothered me before.

I adapted. I began intensive hand and wrist therapy. I learned to use voice recognition software. The university provided a foot-operated mouse. I dictated papers and class assignments. I studied at home using textbooks. Eventually, I began to study lying down on my side, the only position that was comfortable for my back. This, unfortunately, led to neck and shoulder pain.

After completing my board exams (eight hours of sitting down and typing answers to questions on a computer), I was afflicted with excruciating pain for three days. Although school had been challenging until then, I was about to start the most difficult part of medical school, the third year. This entailed long hours caring for patients in the hospital, being on overnight calls without sleep every few days, and studying intensely without much time off.

I knew I couldn't do it. I was in a state of deep despair. Here I was, after getting my degree at Harvard, pursuing my life's passion of studying medicine at one of the top schools in the country, and I had to stop because my body was failing me. I had been in pain for so long that I wondered if it was even possible for me to get better. I had seen some of the top doctors in the country, gotten the best treatments, but continued to decline. I felt hopeless.

I asked for a leave of absence and was granted a year off. I decided I needed to get to the bottom of my illness. Three years of intensive physical therapy, doctor's visits, and medications had not helped at all. Something was missing.

My parents thought diet was a factor. They thought my becoming vegetarian was causing a problem. I believed this was not true because I ate a ton of fruits and vegetables, and ate tofu and dairy products for protein.

I had given up eating meat for ethical, environmental, and spiritual reasons. I was an active member of the San Francisco vegetarian society, had organized vegetarian events for the university, and was a strong advocate for vegetarianism. I thought that my spiritual growth and meditation practice would be deepened by avoiding meat.

I had been studying Ayurveda, the traditional medicine of India, for a while on the side. I decided to visit a practitioner in San Francisco. She diagnosed me with excess vata (air energy) and low ojas (vitality). She recommended some herbs and spices and dietary modifications. She suggested that I eat for my Ayurvedic body type and also incorporate some nourishing foods.

My path to recovery began with two words: bone broth. The Ayurvedic practitioner recommended it as one of the nourishing foods that could help restore vitality in my depleted body. But I was resistant. I could not eat animal products. I went back and forth about this for a few weeks.

Finally, because I was using animal bones that were about to be discarded, I decided that this did not violate my principles. After a month of daily bone broth, I was about 10 percent better, which was the first time anything had helped in years. Bone broth is rich in minerals and gelatin, which support digestive health and help reduce inflammation. My recovery from illness began with healing and repair of my gut.

In the story of the Buddha, after practicing an extreme form of asceticism, the Buddha was weak and near death. He was visited by a milkmaid who offered him a little milk. Despite the taboos against this, he decided to accept and eventually recovered his health. He went on to teach about moderation and the Middle Way. I felt I had reached a similar turning point. I questioned everything I thought I knew about health and disease. I decided to keep an open mind. I realized that there was a lot I didn't know about nutrition and alternative therapies.

Next, I explored acupuncture, visiting three different acupuncturists for ten to twelve sessions each. I didn't see much improvement. I tried qigong. I visited energy healers and Reiki practitioners. I deepened my yoga practice. I continued taking herbs. I improved another 20 percent.

Four months of my year off had passed, and I was still not feeling much better. I was becoming desperate. I decided to experiment with eating meat again. I was deeply conflicted about this after three years of vegetarianism. However, I was willing to try anything to recover my health, because I knew that I could not fulfill my dream of becoming a doctor without a healthy body.

One day I stopped by the UCSF cafeteria and bought a chicken sandwich. I went to an empty classroom where I could eat mindfully. Before eating, I prayed for some sort of sign or clue to let me know if I was doing the right thing.

Eating the sandwich was uneventful. But, as I was chewing the last mouthful of chicken, I bit into something hard. Surprised, I pulled the morsel out of my mouth and realized that it was a tiny rolled-up piece of paper. I unfurled it and saw that it had a word on it. The word was RATION.

I was puzzled. I decided to try to make some sense of this and just think about what the word might mean. To me, a ration was something scarce and valuable consumed during a time of need. Perhaps the message was that I needed a small amount of meat in my diet to get better. To this day, I don't know how that piece of paper got into my sandwich. It's a mystery.

I then meditated on the decision for several days. I realized that perhaps I should try eating meat for a while to see how I felt. My Ayurvedic practitioner agreed with this and explained that certain body types may do better with animal protein. In fact, she had wanted me to eat meat after our first visit. However, she started me initially with bone broths because she sensed I would be more open to that at the beginning, based on my strong ethical convictions.

The improvements were significant. I began eating more protein with each meal and consumed meat regularly. I also ate more eggs. Within two months, I had less pain, had more energy, and had regained some of the weight I had lost.

I then met a holistic chiropractor in Oakland who practiced a form of functional medicine. Although I didn't really understand or believe in what he was doing, at that point I was open to trying anything.

Remarkably, I began to improve right away. The imbalances identified and treated using a functional medicine approach were fundamental to helping me heal fully. Fixing these issues was the final piece of the puzzle. I responded well to holistic chiropractic treatment.

At the end of my year off, all my pain had been resolved. My weight, energy, and mood had normalized. I was able to take a motorcycle trip that I had dreamed about for years. I felt at peace. Interestingly, I did not notice any adverse impact from meat consumption on my meditation and spiritual practice, which was something I had been afraid of. I still had reservations about eating meat but tried to purchase high-quality, organic meats.

I was able to complete medical school and eventually went on to residency at Stanford. I then completed a fellowship in integrative medicine and also decided to learn Ayurveda and functional medicine, the two modalities that helped me the most.

I studied healthy cultures around the world to see what traditional wisdom could teach me. I became a firm believer in the power of nutrition, knowing the impact it had on my life. I learned firsthand about the capacity of the body to heal itself and recover from disease, no matter how bleak things look. Perhaps most important, I developed a strong sense of empathy for my patients, because I had felt the desperation, hopelessness, and despair that one experiences at the lowest points of fighting a chronic illness.

Now, more than ten years later, having helped thousands of patients using these principles, I continue to live my dream of helping people to achieve optimal health using integrative medicine. One of my colleagues, a Feldenkrais practitioner, defines health as the ability to live your dreams. My hope is that by sharing some of the knowledge I have learned from my training and life experience, I can help you to gain the well-being and vitality necessary to pursue your own dreams.

# PART ONE

## Fuel Your Body Optimally

# CHAPTER 1
# HUNTER-GATHERERS AND BLUE ZONES

You may have picked up this book for various reasons. Perhaps you are healthy and looking to maintain your health, or you have certain nonspecific symptoms like fatigue or indigestion, or maybe you have a serious chronic illness and are looking for ways to feel better. In our fast-paced society, optimal health is something that's rather uncommon. This chapter focuses on populations that have actually enjoyed exceptional health and longevity, to see what lessons we can learn from them to incorporate into our own lives.

## Paleo Is a Starting Point

To begin with, let's look at the question, "What is a Paleo diet?" My definition of a Paleo diet is one that you are genetically adapted to eat, based on what your ancestors ate. Now, we are not trying to replicate exactly the diet that your ancestors consumed, because that is not practical. Rather, my goal is to use insights from evolutionary biology and ancestral health principles to inform our modern approach to nutrition. I believe that ultimately Paleo is more of a philosophy and an approach to eating that focuses on the quality of foods rather than getting caught up in the details of different food categories.

Paleo should not be an end point but rather a point of departure to discover your optimal diet. The Paleovedic Diet enables you to customize a Paleo framework using the principles of Ayurveda to determine the diet that is best for you and your unique physiology. Ayurveda states that each person has a unique body type and a particular dietary pattern that is best for him or her. You will discover your body type and learn specific diet and lifestyle recommendations in Chapter 6.

## Why Go Paleo?

Why follow a Paleo diet? The premise is simple. Our human genetic code was basically shaped by the 2.5 million years our ancestors lived as hunter-gatherers, before the advent of agriculture approximately ten thousand years ago. This period of time is known as the Paleolithic era and comprises the vast majority of human history. It's estimated that human beings have lived approximately one hundred thousand generations as hunter-gatherers, compared to about six hundred subsequent generations as farmers.[1] Therefore, for the vast majority of human history, our genes were shaped by the lives our ancestors lived as hunters and gatherers. The agricultural era has had limited effects on our genetic makeup, although there are some interesting initial changes, such as with salivary enzyme levels, as we will discuss later.

British epidemiologist Geoffrey Rose, an expert in public health, explained these ideas in a lucid manner. He wrote that in order to prevent chronic disease, public health officials should recommend removing "unnatural factors" and restoring "'biological normality'—that is, the conditions to which presumably we are genetically adapted."[2] While Rose was referring to factors such as cigarette smoking and physical inactivity, other "unnatural factors" are the industrial processed foods that have appeared in our modern era. The conditions to which we are genetically still adapted are diet and lifestyle patterns that mimic those of our Paleolithic ancestors.

## What the Caveman Really Ate

To determine what exactly human beings ate during the Paleolithic era, scientists have examined the fossil record and also studied modern hunter-gatherer societies. Although the popular perception is that ancestral eating centers on meat consumption, anthropological analysis reveals that some of these populations consume very little meat. For example, the Kitava people from the island of Papua New Guinea consume tubers (sweet potato, yam, and taro), vegetables, fruit, coconut, and fish. They typically consume 70 to 80 percent of calories from carbohydrates. Contrast this with the Inuit Eskimos from Greenland, who consume 70 to 80 percent of calories from fat, mostly saturated fat. Their diet consists of seal, walrus, whale, caribou, fish, and occasionally seaweed.

In 2000, researchers analyzed 229 hunter-gatherer populations that had survived long enough to be studied by anthropologists to determine what type of diet they followed.[3] It was found that these populations consumed animal products whenever possible, and had higher intake of fat and protein and relatively lower intake of carbohydrates (averaging 22 to 40 percent of calories) compared to modern diets. They also preferred fatty animal foods, including organ meats, over the lean muscle meats that we typically find at the grocery store. The wild plant foods they consumed differed from modern carbohydrates in that they were much higher in fiber, higher in nutrients, and lower in simple sugars—they would be very slow to raise blood sugar, causing a correspondingly slow insulin response. As you'll see in Chapter 2, this difference in the type of dietary carbohydrate and the corresponding difference in insulin response is of critical importance.

## Healthy Starches Were Part of the Paleolithic Diet

Scientists have performed sophisticated analyses (using isotope signatures from fossilized bones) and determined that our ancestors also ate roots, tubers, rhizomes, and other underground plant storage organs; it is likely that the consumption of starchy plants goes back at least 250,000 years, well before the advent of agriculture.[4] Therefore, the perception that Paleo is a low-carb, all-meat diet fails to appreciate the fundamental role that healthy starches played in the dietary patterns of our ancestors.

Some of my patients have almost developed a phobia about eating carbohydrates of any type because they have heard many negative ideas about carbs from both mainstream and alternative health sources. There is simply no need for this, because there is nothing intrinsically harmful about carbohydrates. Again, the most important thing is the type and quality of the carbohydrate, which I discuss in detail in Chapter 2. In Chapter 4, I talk much more about wild plant foods that were consumed by our ancestors and provide guidance on how to eat more of these highly nutritious superfoods and their modern descendants.

## Lessons from Weston Price

One of the seminal studies on healthy ancestral populations was conducted by Dr. Weston A. Price, a dentist from Cleveland who practiced during the 1920s. He traveled to hundreds of cities around the world to study populations free of chronic illness and degenerative disease, in places ranging from the Swiss Alps to the Andes Mountains in Peru, multiple locations in Africa, the Polynesian islands, the Arctic, and Australia.[5] As a dentist, Dr. Price's interest was in oral health, and he was surprised to find that there was a remarkable absence of tooth decay and cavities in the people that he visited. This was despite the fact that none of them were brushing their teeth or particularly concerned about their dental hygiene. This led him to believe that dental health was far more closely tied to nutrition than to hygiene.

Dr. Price conducted his research during an era in which modern processed foods were being introduced throughout the world. In population after population, he was able to provide sobering documentation about how the change from a traditional to a modern diet led to dental cavities, negative changes in facial structure, depressed immunity, and other medical problems.[6]

What can we learn about nutrition from these healthy traditional populations? The diets in these "primitive" populations varied tremendously, ranging from 100 percent animal products and seafood among the Inuit Eskimos to fermented whole grains, vegetables, fruits, sweet potatoes, and meat among the native tribes of Africa. However, common features of their diets were whole, unprocessed foods, an abundance of fats—especially animal fats—from dairy products and meat, seafood and animal protein when available (especially organ meats), and certain raw plant foods. Some of the diets included seeds, grains, and nuts, but these were typically prepared by soaking, sprouting, fermentation, or other traditional preparation methods that made them easily digestible. There was also a notable absence of modern foods like white sugar, white flour, vegetable oils, and other processed foods.

## The Blue Zones—Lessons for Living Longer

Let's fast-forward eighty years to modern times. Researchers have identified a few areas in today's world known as "blue zones," where populations still enjoy exceptional longevity and good health (but don't follow a hunter-gatherer lifestyle).[7] These include Okinawa, Japan (where people enjoy the longest life expectancy in the world), Loma Linda, California (where the population lives about ten years longer than other Americans), Ikaria, Greece (where nearly one in three people make it to their nineties), and Nicoya, Costa Rica. Remarkably, all of these different populations appear to enjoy excellent health and are less affected by the common chronic illnesses prevalent in modern society. Let us take a quick look at these blue zones to see what we can learn from these unique groups.

Some factors are common to people in all blue zones. These include regular physical activity that is incorporated into daily living, a whole-foods plant-based diet incorporating homegrown fruits and vegetables, strong social connections with friends and family, and a sense of purpose and meaning in life. Other aspects are unique to particular populations. For example, in Okinawa, Japan, a plant-based diet rich in vegetables, sweet potatoes, and tofu coupled with homegrown spices such as mugwort, ginger, and turmeric provides powerful nutritional support; a clear sense of purpose, termed *ikigai*, or "reason for waking up in the morning," is important to elders in Okinawa.[8] Another unique practice commonly followed in Okinawa is *hara hachi bu*, which means to stop eating when your stomach is about 80 percent full—a beneficial practice to prevent overeating and limit portion size.[9] Of note, Ayurveda also recommends eating until you're about two thirds full.

In Loma Linda, California, the Seventh-Day Adventist population is one of the few blue zones in the United States, with studies showing that typical life expectancy is seven or eight years longer than in other parts of California; Adventists are often vegetarian or consume meat only rarely, but consume a nutrient-rich plant-based diet incorporating fruits, vegetables, legumes, and nuts of different types.[10] They also incorporate a weekly break during the Sabbath on weekends when they spend time with family and friends and focus on rest and rejuvenation.

In Nicoya, Costa Rica, strong social networks and a focus on family is coupled with a strong sense of purpose known as *plan de vida*; like many other blue zone populations, Nicoyans get most of their calories during the daytime and eat a light dinner.[11]

In Ikaria, Greece, there are a number of different factors that contribute to a social environment that promotes longevity. These include very strong social connections, a diet rich in fruits, vegetables, and legumes, daily wine consumption, low stress levels, plenty of rest (incorporating a daily afternoon nap), and regular physical activity. Daily moderate consumption of alcohol, such as a serving or two of red wine, is an attribute of Ikarian society that is common in other blue zones as well.

It is important to realize that there is no one magic bullet that explains longevity in each of these countries. What matters is the synergistic combination of multiple factors that contribute to create an ecosystem of health and longevity around each person.[12]

## Eat Anything You Want—Except a Western Diet

The reality is that healthy ancestral populations varied widely in the types of diets they ate and the level of carbohydrates in their diet—but they were still healthier overall. Clearly it is possible for humans to be healthy while following a wide range of diet types. Whenever specific populations deviate from their traditional diets, whatever their traditional diets might be, their rates of obesity and illness appear to increase. Human beings can thrive and be free of disease on a wide variety of different diets—except the modern Western diet. I should clarify that by "Western diet" I mean a diet that features substantial amounts of refined grains, vegetables oils, sweetened beverages, white flour, and sweets.

Once people eat a Western diet, they get Western diseases, especially obesity, diabetes, heart disease, and cancer. For example, women in Japan have one of the lowest breast cancer rates in the world, but when these women emigrate to the United States, in just two generations their descendants experienced the same increased breast cancer rates as other Americans.[13] Similar trends for breast cancer have been observed among the Inuit Eskimos and Native Americans. The same applies for other types of cancer and other common Western diseases. People within the same ethnic population get more modern diseases when they move to more urban or Western locations; this well-established fact demonstrates the deleterious effects of modern dietary staples such as processed sugars, flour, and refined grains.[14]

In Okinawa, increasing adoption of a Western diet, including processed foods and fast foods, has led to a sharp increase in obesity and related diseases, such as diabetes; the life expectancy of men in Okinawa has also dropped significantly, especially among the younger generation, who are not adhering to the strict diet and lifestyle patterns of their long-lived elders.[15]

The take-home lesson here is that eating nutrient-dense whole foods promotes health. Eating nutrient-poor, calorie-rich foods, especially those with easily digested simple carbohydrates, promotes high insulin levels, which lead to obesity, inflammation, and associated chronic diseases. Maximizing nutrient density in your diet essentially means eating whole foods and avoiding processed or industrialized foods, especially sugar and white flour.

In addition to eating what your ancestors might have eaten, it is equally important and perhaps more so *to not eat foods that were not part of their traditional diets*. The goal is to minimize calorie-rich, nutrient-poor foods such as highly processed grains, refined flour, sweetened beverages, vegetable oils, refined sugar, and candy—foods that your ancestors did not have access to as recently as two hundred years ago.

## The Power of Social Connection

One thing that strikes me the most about the people who live in blue zones is their commitment to cultivating social connections and the tremendous value they place on family and friends. When you read about the daily lives of these people, it's interesting to note that many of them spend literally a few hours almost every single day in relaxed, quality time with family, neighbors, and friends. That level of intense interconnectedness is in stark contrast to the epidemic of isolation and disconnectedness that so many people in the West suffer from. Although it is difficult to calculate exactly what percentage social connections contribute to the longevity of these populations, there is no doubt in my mind that it plays a huge role.

One simple thing that you can do to start emulating these long-lived communities is to cultivate more richness and more depth in your social relationships. There many different ways to do this, even if you are single or live alone:

- join a group
- take some classes
- get to know your neighbors
- reconnect with old friends
- deepen your relationships with your loved ones
- make an effort to get to know coworkers
- volunteer in any setting that you enjoy
- get a pet
- connect with others online
- set an intention to strengthen your social connections

# CHAPTER 2

# CARBS, GRAINS, AND GLUTEN

Carbohydrates are probably the most debated aspect of any modern diet. How much do you need? What types of carbs are best, and in what proportion at each meal? This chapter is a primer on the essentials of carbohydrate consumption. Carbohydrates have an important role in providing energy, antioxidants, vitamins, minerals, and fiber; they can help raise levels of the beneficial neurotransmitter serotonin, but can also raise levels of insulin if consumed in excess. I clarify which carbohydrates are best, how much you need, and how to consume carbohydrates while avoiding harmful effects on insulin and other hormones.

The Paleovedic Diet is not opposed to the consumption of carbohydrates. On the contrary, healthy starches are an essential dietary staple for almost everyone. Healthy starches for all people include vegetables, fruits, and tubers. Healthy starches for some people, depending on their tolerance, include legumes, nuts, seeds, and possibly certain grains. There may be certain situations during which diets lower in carbohydrates may be preferable, but I don't recommend a low carbohydrate diet for all people. I also find from my patients' experience, especially within the Paleo community, that people are often consuming far fewer carbohydrates than they realize. This can be harmful for health in a number of ways, for example, by being too low in the beneficial carbohydrates necessary to support healthy gut flora.

## Simple vs. Complex Carbs

As we saw in Chapter 1, the difference between ancestral diets and modern diets is the type and quality of the carbohydrates consumed. Ancestral diets usually had nutrient-dense, low-glycemic carbohydrates. These include vegetables, fruits, nuts, seeds, tubers, and other plant parts. Notably, they did not include sugar or white flour. In contrast, modern diets feature nutrient-poor, high-glycemic carbohydrates such as most breads, pasta, pizza, sweetened beverages, beer, and candy. The fundamental difference between these two types of carbohydrate is their effect on insulin.

This ties in to my definition of the difference between simple and complex carbohydrates. Simple carbohydrates include most sugars that are broken down and absorbed quickly, such as white sugar, jams, jellies, corn syrup, candy, and sweetened beverages. Honey, unrefined maple syrup, and molasses are examples of simple carbohydrates that are relatively less processed and contain beneficial vitamins and minerals and therefore can be enjoyed in moderation. Complex carbohydrates include starches and longer-chain molecules that are broken down more slowly, such as vegetables of all kinds, beans, and legumes, and properly cooked and prepared whole grains.

Among simple carbohydrates, fructose (like in high-fructose corn syrup) is especially problematic because it is processed by the liver. Known by biochemists as "the most lipogenic carbohydrate," fructose is the carbohydrate that is most effective at lipogenesis, the creation of body fat—in other words, it is the type of carbohydrate that your body most readily converts into fat.[1] Now, many types of fruit contain fructose, but it is combined with vitamins, minerals, antioxidants, and fiber and therefore well-balanced as a whole food. Therefore, fructose in fruits is not harmful in moderation, unlike fructose in processed foods and sweetened beverages.

## Quantify Carbs with Glycemic Index and Glycemic Load

The distinction between simple and complex carbohydrates is not as helpful as the concept of the glycemic index (GI), which enables quantification of the effect of foods on blood sugar. The glycemic index refers to how quickly your blood sugar rises when you consume a particular food. It is a scale that goes from 0 to 100, with 100 being white sugar. It is only relevant to carbohydrates, as foods that are mostly protein or fat, such as meat and fish, do not have a major effect on blood sugar. Simple carbohydrates have a higher glycemic index, and complex carbohydrates have a lower glycemic index. Foods with a higher GI tend to raise blood sugar more rapidly, followed by a swift decline or "crash," while foods with a lower GI produce a gradual, relatively low rise in blood sugar that remains stable.

An additional fundamental concept is the glycemic load (GL). GL is derived from glycemic index but also factors in the amount of carbohydrates in each food and what the typical serving size is, thereby offering a more "real-life" measure of the effect of a particular food on blood sugar. For example, we typically consume a larger quantity of potatoes in an average serving when compared to fruit, and this is factored into the glycemic load calculations.

You want to minimize foods that have a glycemic index over 50 or a glycemic load over 20.

**Table 1: Glycemic Index vs. Glycemic Load**

| Glycemic Category | Glycemic Index | Glycemic Load |
|---|---|---|
| Low | <30 | <10 |
| Medium | 31 to 50 | 11 to 20 |
| High | >50 | >20 |

Let's look at some actual values from the scientific literature.[2,3] Vegetables such as carrots (GL 2), pumpkins (GL 3), beets (GL 4), and green peas (GL 4) have a low glycemic load. Leafy green vegetables have a negligible effect on blood sugar and an extremely low glycemic load. Fruits, although usually medium or high in terms of glycemic index, tend to have a low glycemic load—for example, strawberries (GL 1), oranges (GL 5), and watermelon (GL 4). Legumes also tend to score low on the scale—black beans, lentils, and mung beans all have a GL of 5. Nuts are low glycemic, for example, cashews (GL 3) and peanuts (GL 1).

Dairy products such as yogurt also have a low GL, with plain yogurt scoring lower than those with flavors or added fruits. Processed grains like bagels (GL 24), cereals such as cornflakes (GL 23), and foods made from refined flour tend to rank higher on the scale. In contrast, oatmeal (GL 10) and granola (GL 7) have relatively lower glycemic loads and would therefore be better options, although note that instant oatmeal has a much higher GL of 30. Dried fruits such as dates (GL 18) and raisins (GL 28) tend to rank higher than their fresh counterparts.

In terms of root vegetables, potatoes vary depending on how they are prepared. Boiled (GL 16) and mashed (GL 17) tend to have a lower glycemic load than baked potatoes (GL 33). An excellent way to improve the glycemic index of potatoes is to chill them in the refrigerator for twenty-four hours after cooking them by any method. This transforms the starch in the potatoes to "resistant starch," which has a lower glycemic index and also is beneficial for your gut bacteria, as discussed in Chapter 5.[4] After you have chilled the potatoes for twenty-four hours, you can either have them cold as in a potato salad, or you can reheat them, and the resistant starch will remain intact, maintaining the lower glycemic properties—these potatoes have a GL of about 8. The addition of a vinaigrette dressing (containing olive oil and vinegar) further reduces the glycemic load of chilled potatoes. The effect of vinegar in this case is likely due to its acid content, so other high-acid foods such as tomato juice, lime juice, lemon juice, or apple cider vinegar should probably work as well. So enjoy your potatoes, but simply chill them and slather them with olive oil and vinegar!

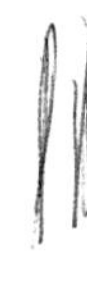

Sweet potatoes, which are lower glycemic than white potatoes, also have a different GL depending on how they are cooked. Boiled or steamed sweet potatoes have a low glycemic load of about 11 compared to a baked sweet potato, which has a GL of 42. This is because the starches are broken down in different ways depending on the cooking method. Steaming would be preferable to boiling because water-soluble nutrients could be lost in the boiling water if you discard it after cooking.

As for grains, the more processed and refined a grain is, the higher the glycemic load. For example, white rice (GL 23) ranks higher than brown rice (GL 18), and white bread (GL 11–12) higher than wheat bread (GL 8). However, white rice is one of the easiest grains to digest, so in moderation it can be part of a healthy diet; this speaks to the broader issue that other factors besides glycemic index must be considered in the evaluation of each food. Moreover, a special method of preparing white rice reduces its calories and leads to the formation of resistant starch, which is lower glycemic and has beneficial effects on gut bacteria (this method is discussed in chapter 5). With pasta, just as with potatoes, the cooking method affects glycemic performance. If pasta is cooked al dente, where it is still a little bit firm and chewy, it has a lower glycemic load (GL 19) than pasta that is cooked completely until soft (GL 29).

As a rule of thumb, consuming foods with a GL less than 20 is preferable for maintaining healthy blood sugar. This does not mean that you could never eat foods that have a higher glycemic load—it just means that you have to be extra careful with portion size. For example, a small quantity of raisins or a couple of dates, even though they have a GL >20, can comprise a nutritious part of a healthy snack or meal.

## Eat Protein and Fat Every Time You Eat Carbs

Food combinations affect how quickly a meal raises blood sugar. Consuming significant quantities of protein, good fats, and fiber along with carbohydrates slows down the digestion and absorption of the carbohydrates, thereby lowering the glycemic index of the meal. For example, a plain pizza with Parmesan cheese and tomato sauce has a high GI of 80 and a GL of 22. In contrast, a supreme pizza with meat, vegetables, and cheese has a significantly lower GI of 36 and GL of 9 (not that I'm recommending that you eat a supreme pizza every day!). Another study evaluated the addition of certain toppings, such as baked beans, chili con carne, tuna, and cheddar cheese, to the carb-heavy foods pasta, white potatoes, and wheat bread; it found that the added toppings, especially cheddar cheese and tuna, consistently lowered the glycemic index of all three carbohydrate-rich foods.[5]

Perhaps you're wondering why this is the case. One reason relates to gastric emptying, which is how quickly the stomach empties its contents into the small intestine after a meal. The faster the stomach empties, the more quickly the digested food goes into the intestine, where it can be absorbed and consequently raise blood sugar. The addition of fat slows down gastric emptying, thereby slowing down the release of food into the intestine and also the absorption into the blood of the carbohydrates consumed. With protein, part of its impact comes from stimulation of additional insulin secretion, which helps to process the additional blood sugar and drives the absorbed sugar more rapidly and efficiently into the cells.[6] Most likely other mechanisms are involved as well, but several studies have demonstrated that the addition of protein and fat to a carbohydrate-containing meal lowers the overall glycemic index of the meal in a healthy person.[7]

This is why I recommend eating adequate amounts of protein, good fats, and fiber with every meal or snack. The reason I am emphasizing these macronutrients and not suggesting that you focus on getting adequate carbohydrates is that most foods contain some quantity of carbohydrates. To reiterate, it is ideal to try to incorporate protein and fat along with your carbohydrates *every time you eat.* Protein, fats, and fiber are also the key elements that make you feel full and satiated, which is another reason they are so important.

Ayurveda emphasizes the importance of not combining certain incompatible foods. For example, it has been said that fruit should always be eaten by itself on an empty stomach. I respectfully disagree with this particular Ayurvedic rule about food combinations. The stated reason is that fruit is digested very quickly and should therefore not be combined with other foods that take more time to digest. However, this is exactly the reason fruit should be combined with other foods such as protein and fat whenever possible. This ensures that the carbohydrates in the fruit are broken down and absorbed more slowly, thereby lowering the glycemic index of the fruit.

## Remarkable Benefits of a Low-glycemic Diet

A low-glycemic diet has been shown to be a strong predictor of future health, as people on a low GI diet tend to have a reduced risk of diabetes, heart disease, and certain cancers.[8] Consuming a high-glycemic diet appears to increase the risk of weight gain and obesity. In a ten-year study involving more than seventy-five thousand women, those who were eating a high-glycemic diet were the most likely to develop heart disease.[9] In addition, a high-glycemic diet appears to increase the risk of gallbladder disease.[10] Low-glycemic diets have been shown to be beneficial in patients with hyperlipidemia, diabetes, and obesity, probably as a result of improving insulin sensitivity.[11] Therefore, the evidence is clear that a low glycemic index is one critical quality of a healthy diet.

As discussed above, adding fat and protein to carbohydrates is one proven way to reduce the glycemic index of meals. This is why I don't believe in overzealous recommendations of low-fat diets for everyone. Removing the beneficial fats, in addition to having other detrimental effects, takes away a key macronutrient that can help reduce the overall glycemic index of the person's diet.

Vegetables, meat and fish, nuts, legumes, dairy products, and most fruits have a low glycemic load. Not coincidentally, these are the main types of foods that I recommend as part of the Paleovedic Diet, which is a naturally low-glycemic diet. For a complete list of the glycemic index and glycemic load of various foods, please visit my website.

## Carbohydrate Density Is Another Useful Marker

In addition to glycemic index and load, there is another concept that can be used to evaluate carbohydrates, known as carbohydrate density. This can be defined as the number of grams of carbohydrate per 100 g of a food. Most carbohydrate-containing foods consumed by traditional populations, such as vegetables, tubers, fruits, and nuts, are much lower in carbohydrate density than modern foods like grains, sugar, refined flour, and other processed foods. One paper hypothesizes that this lower carbohydrate density has a beneficial effect on the intestinal microbiome, which reduces inflammation and may positively affect metabolic hormones such as leptin.[12] The Paleovedic Diet naturally includes foods with low carbohydrate density.

## Limitations of Glycemic Index and Glycemic Load

There are some limitations to the concepts of glycemic index and load. The main one is that it does not consider differences between individuals. One of the key tenets of Ayurveda is that every person is unique, and each person's response to carbohydrates can be slightly different. Genetic differences in insulin production may partially explain these differences. Research conducted by Stanford Professor Gerald Reaven, a diabetes researcher who has been studying insulin resistance since 1968, has shed light on this.[13]

Dr. Reaven found that people's insulin responses to carbohydrates are quite varied—two healthy people without any diagnosable blood sugar problem, when consuming an identical quantity of the same food, may have very different subsequent changes in their insulin and blood sugar levels.[14] In approximately 25 percent of a normal population, insulin response to carbohydrates is blunted. When these people eat excess carbohydrates, their insulin levels do not rapidly surge upward. On the other hand, 25 percent of people have an elevated insulin response to carbohydrates, therefore responding in a very different way to the same carbohydrate intake. The other 50 percent of people are somewhere in between—not as elevated as the 25 percent who have a high response, but still quite significant. Why does this matter? First of all, elevated insulin levels lead to fat accumulation in our adipose tissue. Chronic or recurrent elevation in serum insulin will promote weight gain through fat accretion.

The second reason has to do with glycemic index and glycemic load. These values are established by measuring the blood sugar in a group of test subjects (at least six to eight people) after consuming a certain food *and then calculating the average of all the results*. Usually each individual ends up with a different number, and the average of the values is defined as the GI. Different studies evaluating the same quantity of the same food have led to different numbers for the GI. These studies are done in "healthy" people without diabetes but do not take into account the variable insulin response of each individual. Each person who is consuming a specific food may have a different blood sugar response—and potentially a different GI for the same food.

Now, this does not mean that these concepts are useless. We just have to remember that, like other concepts, glycemic index and load have their limitations and must be individualized for your particular body type and physiology.

## My Experience with Carbs

My own experience with carbohydrates has been interesting. Over the years, I have cultivated the ability to assess the effects of food on my body relatively quickly. For better or for worse, I react pretty quickly to foods and have learned to interpret the signals my body gives me. I can tell based on energy levels and various aches and pains if I have consumed too much carbohydrate.

Over time, I have noticed that my tolerance of carbohydrates has decreased, although my level of physical activity has been the same. This may be partially because of a strong family history of diabetes, which unfortunately is epidemic among Indian-Americans. I have gradually reduced the quantity of carbohydrates in my diet and eliminated all grains about a year ago. I continue to thrive on root vegetables like sweet potatoes, carrots, beets, cassava, yucca, and taro.

Even white rice, a grain that I have consumed my whole life, is something that I don't tolerate well anymore. Therefore, I have given it up, except for the occasional *dosa* (a crepe made from fermented white rice and lentils). Even though white rice is comparable in glycemic index to root vegetables such as sweet potatoes, I feel noticeably worse when I eat rice. This may have something to do with the relatively higher carbohydrate density of grains such as rice when compared to root vegetables. As we discussed above, root vegetables (and all other components of a Paleo diet) tend to be significantly lower in carbohydrate density than cereal grains, including rice.

## Insulin Drives Weight Gain and Obesity

We have learned a great deal about the fundamental role of hormones such as insulin in metabolic imbalances. Abnormal insulin patterns play a primary role in blood sugar dysregulation, weight gain, and obesity. As Harvard Medical School Professor George Cahill put it, "Carbohydrate is driving insulin is driving fat."[15] High insulin levels, produced by our modern high-glycemic high-carbohydrate diet, promote the deposition and buildup of fat in our fat cells and tissues. This dramatic shift in the type of carbohydrates that we consume is largely responsible for the obesity epidemic.

## Insulin Promotes Inflammation

What you may not know is the role of insulin in inflammation. It is believed that silent inflammation is the root cause of most modern Western diseases, such as heart disease, cancer, dementia, and stroke. You may not even know that you have silent inflammation until one of these diseases strikes. This is another reason why it makes sense to optimize your insulin levels.

## Insulin Resistance and Blood Sugar Dysregulation

Insulin resistance, where the body doesn't respond to insulin as it should, is present in diabetes (afflicting 26 million Americans) and is also the hallmark of metabolic syndrome, a metabolic disorder affecting 47 million Americans. In addition, almost 79 million Americans have prediabetes, abnormal blood sugar that is not yet high enough to qualify as diabetes. We have an epidemic of blood sugar imbalance in the United States, and it's only getting worse: the Centers for Disease Control and Prevention (CDC), the federal agency in charge of public health, estimates that children born today have a lifetime risk of developing diabetes of 1 in 3.

## High Insulin May Increase Your Risk of Cancer

Research suggests that there may be a link between elevated insulin levels and cancer. A number of studies postulate a link between elevated blood levels of insulin and the development and progression of various types of cancer, especially colon, breast, pancreatic, and prostate.[16] While more research is needed to investigate this connection, it's beneficial to try to get your insulin level down to the optimal range.

## How Many Carbs Should You Eat?

Optimal carbohydrate intake can vary widely depending on age, metabolism, activity level, and other factors. I consider a low-carbohydrate diet to consist of less than 10 percent of calories from carbs, moderate to be between 10 and 40 percent, and high-carbohydrate to be more than 40 percent of calories from carbs. While the total number of carbs depends on your caloric requirements, low-carb is typically under 50 g of carbohydrates per day, assuming a 2,000-calorie daily diet. The standard American diet can easily include more than 300 g of carbohydrates per day, which is excessive. The most important element is to focus on the type and quality of your carbs, which should be primarily from vegetables, fruits, legumes, and perhaps some gluten-free grains.

One marker that can be useful is your fasting insulin level, which is not perfect but can provide helpful information about your metabolic status. For example, one study found that a fasting insulin level of 12 was associated with a three-fold higher incidence of prediabetes than a fasting insulin level of 5.[17] It is possible for someone to have an elevated fasting insulin level but still have a normal fasting blood sugar. Therefore, I suggest that during your annual physical you ask your doctor to order a fasting insulin level, in addition to the usual fasting blood sugar, cholesterol, and other lab tests. While most labs have different reference ranges for normal insulin, the following general guidelines may be useful:

**Table 2: Fasting Insulin Level**

| Category | Fasting insulin (uIU/mL) |
|---|---|
| Optimal | <5 |
| Normal | 5–10 |
| High | >10 |

Trying to optimize your insulin level has significant benefits. If it is above 10, I would suggest following the Paleovedic Diet for two months and then rechecking. If it is still elevated, then try to increase physical activity as much as possible. If that does not lower it enough, I would incorporate intermittent fasting, which I cover in Chapter 8. Please work with your physician or nutritionist as you make such changes.

## Removing Refined Carbs Helps Everyone

You might wonder why certain people still lose weight on a high-carb, low-fat diet. The likely explanation is that even in a low-fat diet, refined carbohydrates, which are the most fattening, are still reduced. Therefore, such people probably lose weight more because of what they are not eating than what they are eating. Even the very low–fat diet (10 percent calories from fat) publicized by Dr. Dean Ornish restricts all refined carbohydrates—no sugar, white rice, or white flour. Removing these refined carbohydrates takes out the most fattening component in most people's diets.

Incidentally, refined carbs are the explanation behind the well-established correlation between poverty and obesity. One might think that people who are poor can afford less food and are therefore less likely to be obese. In fact, the opposite is true. Populations throughout the world tend to be obese in direct proportion to how poor they are.[18] There was a fascinating study that analyzed overweight women in poor urban areas in the developing world. It found that the poorest women were often the most overweight. The reason for this is the type of food being consumed, an issue of quality rather than quantity. The least expensive foods include refined carbohydrates, bread, white flour, sugar, and processed carbohydrates, which often make up the majority of the diet consumed by poor populations. These foods are calorie rich but nutrient poor, leading to the coexistence of obesity and malnutrition.

## Non-Celiac Gluten Sensitivity

Wheat may be the most controversial carbohydrate, especially because of a protein in wheat known as gluten. There is much debate about whether gluten sensitivity even exists, but from my clinical experience with patients, I am confident that it does. Gluten sensitivity is part of a spectrum, with celiac disease on one end and mild gluten sensitivity on the other. Patients with mild gluten sensitivity may test negative using traditional blood tests for celiac disease but still experience silent inflammation and harmful effects from consuming wheat. In the medical world, this is called non-celiac gluten sensitivity (NCGS). Possible symptoms reported in the literature include abdominal pain, rashes, eczema, headache, "foggy mind," fatigue, diarrhea, mood changes, arm or leg numbness, and joint pain.

In my integrative medicine practice, I have found gluten sensitivity to be associated with a variety of disorders, including autism, allergies, irritable bowel syndrome, ADHD, depression, chronic migraines, and a variety of autoimmune diseases, including Hashimoto's disease, rheumatoid arthritis, psoriasis, and ulcerative colitis. Obviously, this does not mean that every person with these issues is suffering from gluten sensitivity, but it is something worth thinking about in people with such conditions.

Besides gluten, there are several other proteins in wheat that may be problematic, such as three different types of gliadin, lectins such as wheat germ agglutinin (WGA), and pest resistance molecules known as alpha-amylase/trypsin inhibitors (ATIs).[19] So it's possible that people may have reactions to other components of wheat besides gluten. Moreover, wheat is part of a class of foods known as FODMAPs that bother many patients with irritable bowel syndrome.

FODMAP stands for fermentable, oligo-, di-, mono-saccharides and polyols. Foods that contain FODMAPs, such as wheat, have certain carbohydrates that are poorly absorbed and pass into the large intestine where they are fermented by bacteria. Examples of foods high in FODMAPs are grains such as wheat, barley, and rye; vegetables such as asparagus, onion, garlic, and cauliflower; high-lactose dairy such as milk and cottage cheese; and fruits such as apple, banana, and watermelon. For detailed recommendations on how to follow a low-FODMAP diet, please visit my website.

It is clear that the effects of wheat on the body are mediated by a variety of different compounds and cannot be attributed only to gluten. Perhaps we have focused too much on gluten, which does not capture all the physiological effects of a complex whole food like wheat. However, for the sake of simplicity in this book, I use the term *gluten sensitivity* since that is the term that is in the literature now, although perhaps *wheat sensitivity* may be a more accurate term.

As mentioned above, FODMAP-containing foods selectively feed the growth of bacteria in the intestine; therefore, if a person has bacterial imbalances such as small intestinal bacterial overgrowth (SIBO) or bacterial dysbiosis, then a low-FODMAP diet would help. Bacterial dysbiosis is defined in the scientific literature as "qualitative and quantitative changes in the gastrointestinal flora, their metabolic activities, and/or their local distribution that produces harmful effects on the host"; it has been associated with irritable bowel syndrome as well as other conditions, such as eczema, inflammatory bowel disease, and rheumatoid arthritis.[20] There are many different types of dysbiosis—some subtypes that I see in my practice include low levels or poor diversity of beneficial bacteria, overgrowth of pathogenic bacteria or yeast, improper metabolic functions of gut bacteria, or the presence of bacteria in large numbers in places where they are not supposed to be (such as the small intestine).

Just as reported in the medical literature, many of my patients with irritable bowel syndrome suffer from dysbiosis, and the low-FODMAP diet begins to treat this by reducing levels of pathogenic bacteria. In fact, studies have shown that such a diet is a beneficial first-line therapy in patients with irritable bowel syndrome.[21]

One controversial study suggested that because patients with non-celiac gluten sensitivity do well on a low-FODMAP diet, their real issue is not gluten but rather FODMAP sensitivity.[22] I have heard some practitioners say that this study proves that gluten sensitivity does not exist and that NCGS is in reality just a sensitivity to FODMAPs. I do not believe this is accurate. First, the study used whey protein as a negative control, assuming that patients with gluten sensitivity should do fine on whey protein and should not have any reaction to it. The study concluded that because patients had equal worsening of symptoms on gluten and whey protein, there were no gluten-specific effects.

In my clinical practice, patients who are sensitive to gluten are also often sensitive to dairy. Therefore, it is not a valid assumption that dairy proteins can be a good negative control in such patients. Moreover, since wheat, barley, and rye are FODMAPs, following a low-FODMAP diet effectively involves eliminating gluten—it is not surprising that this would benefit patients with non-celiac gluten sensitivity.

In my experience, non-celiac gluten sensitivity is a very real and legitimate condition, distinct from FODMAP sensitivity, which often relates to imbalances in gut bacteria, such as small intestinal bacterial overgrowth (SIBO) or bacterial dysbiosis. Patients with NCGS may commonly have bacterial imbalances such as SIBO, and, therefore, a low-FODMAP diet may be initially beneficial for them. However, the low-FODMAP diet will not offer a permanent cure unless the underlying digestive imbalances are addressed.

## Addiction to Wheat Is Biochemical

When wheat is digested in the body, certain compounds known as gluten exorphins (sometimes called gluteomorphins) are produced; interestingly, dairy products under certain conditions can also lead to the production of similar compounds known as casein exorphins.[23] These chemicals cross the blood-brain barrier, enter the brain, and bind to the same receptors that bind opiates like morphine and heroin, triggering a mild euphoria.[24] Therefore, when my patients tell me that they are addicted to wheat, I know that there is a very real physiological mechanism behind this addiction. In fact, when someone eliminates gluten, they can sometimes go through an uncomfortable withdrawal period just like people with other addictions when they stop using what they are addicted to. The good news is that withdrawal from wheat addiction is less painful and shorter in duration than withdrawal from opiate drugs.

## Celiac Disease Has Become Much More Prevalent

In the last fifty years, there has been a dramatic increase in gluten sensitivity and celiac disease; for example, comparison with old stored blood samples shows an alarming 500 percent increase in the incidence of celiac disease over the last fifty years.[25] Certainly, there is an increased awareness of celiac disease, and testing is much more common, although even today perhaps only a fifth of people who have celiac disease actually know that they have it. However, there are two important factors that have contributed to a real rise in the prevalence of this condition.

## Changes in the Microbiome Predispose to Gluten Sensitivity

The human microbiome, which consists of approximately 100 trillion bacteria per person, has been significantly changing over the past several decades. There is a growing body of research elucidating the vital roles of our gut bacteria in many aspects of health. Factors such as changing diets and the increased use of antibiotics have led to declines in gut bacteria that may be contributing to the increase in gluten sensitivity. The deterioration of our microbiota is potentially linked to the dramatic increase in the incidence of allergies and sensitivities to both foods and environmental triggers.

Taking antibiotics later on during our adult lives could possibly precipitate the development of celiac disease. A large Swedish study analyzing thousands of people diagnosed with celiac disease found that these individuals were more likely than healthy control subjects to have taken antibiotics within the preceding several months.[26] Interestingly, the risk increased in proportion to the number of courses of antibiotics a person was prescribed; the drug metronidazole, which is a broad-spectrum antibiotic that disrupts flora, had the highest association with celiac disease.[27] This is only correlation, and correlation does not imply causation; we cannot say that taking antibiotics caused the person to develop celiac disease. However, it is a provocative finding, and it will be interesting to follow this research as it evolves.

Traditional populations that were healthy and tolerated wheat well differed from us in that they also had all of the factors that would contribute to a robust microbiome, such as regular consumption of fermented foods, exposure to a variety of microbes through farming and close contact with animals, lack of antibiotic use, and so forth. The microbiome is discussed in detail in Chapter 5.

## Not Your Grandmother's Wheat

A secondary factor in the rise of gluten sensitivity has to do with the food supply. Genetic modification and selective breeding to increase crop yields over the years has dramatically changed the genetics and chemical composition of wheat.

The type of wheat that we currently consume is called dwarf wheat, named for its short stature relative to other varietals of wheat. Despite its diminutive size, dwarf wheat is highly prolific and produces a lot more grains per acre, which is an outstanding trait for productivity and profitability.[28] However, its nutritional content has declined over the years—ancient grains such as einkorn wheat are 200 to 400 percent higher in vitamin A, vitamin E, and the antioxidant lutein as well as certain minerals when compared to modern wheat.[29] Dwarf wheat is also significantly higher in starch content, especially in a type of starch called amylopectin A that contributes to a higher glycemic index for wheat and has been associated with insulin resistance.[30]

Unfortunately, it is much higher in gluten than older strains of wheat; modern wheat has up to forty times as much gluten as wheat from earlier this century.[31] Moreover, the types of gluten present in the wheat also were transformed. Specifically, modern wheat contains high levels of an allergenic gluten protein known as glia-$\alpha$9, which is notably absent in ancient grains; interestingly, most patients with celiac disease react negatively to glia-$\alpha$9.[32]

## Genetically Engineered Wheat

The genetic engineering performed to create dwarf wheat also resulted in a plant with extra sets of chromosomes, encoding new proteins with unpredictable effects in humans.[33] Dwarf wheat has forty-two chromosomes (known as hexaploid), unlike einkorn wheat, possibly the oldest form of cultivated wheat, which has a simple genetic structure of fourteen chromosomes (known as diploid).[34] The significance of this is that modern wheat has a lot more genes encoding more proteins than any grain that our bodies are used to encountering and processing. Interestingly, one study showed that unmodified ancient grains such as einkorn wheat may be better tolerated by people with celiac disease (although, of course, I recommend that patients with celiac disease do not consume any type of wheat).[35] Suffice it to say that the wheat that's available today is very different from the wheat that your grandmother may have used to bake bread.

There may be differences from country to country in terms of wheat varietals, processing techniques, and so forth. Some of my patients report that they tolerate wheat in other parts of the world (e.g., the Middle East and, to a lesser degree, Europe) much better than they tolerate wheat in the United States—in fact, some of them cannot have wheat at all in the United States but can have it with impunity in certain other countries. It is not clear what is responsible for these differences. Perhaps it has something do with different species of wheat, genetic modification, method of processing within the food industry, variations in pesticides applied to wheat, or other factors.

To summarize, modern wheat has much more gluten, different types of gluten that people are more sensitive to, far more new genetic material, higher starch content, and lower levels of vitamins, minerals, and antioxidants when compared to ancient wheat. During the last half-century, our human DNA has not experienced major changes commensurate with this radical transformation of wheat, and many people's bodies simply may not be capable of processing modern wheat effectively. Add to this the unprecedented alteration of the human microbiota, and you have a perfect storm of criteria that have contributed to striking increases in celiac disease and gluten sensitivity.

## Certain People Can Eat Wheat and Be Healthy

This is not to say that there aren't certain people who could eat ancient strains of wheat under certain conditions and be healthy. There have been healthy traditional cultures that consumed wheat. For example, Weston Price noted certain populations, such as people in Switzerland, who regularly ate wheat and had excellent health overall. I should reiterate that traditional populations that were healthy and consumed wheat also had the often undervalued characteristics that would contribute to a healthy microbiome, such as consumption of fermented foods, exposure to a variety of microbes through farming and close contact with animals, and paucity of antibiotic use. The robustness and strength of their microbiome made a significant difference in being able to tolerate wheat.

In addition, traditional populations used older, unmodified strains of wheat and utilized stone-ground whole wheat berries rather than refined white flour. They also fermented their wheat before consumption. Of note, wheat that is prepared in such a traditional manner, such as sourdough bread that has undergone a long fermentation, has been found to contain much less gluten than traditional wheat.[36] Moreover, one study that had patients with celiac disease consume properly fermented sourdough bread (which was found to contain less than 10 parts per million of gluten) for sixty days found that there was no adverse effect on clinical symptoms or intestinal pathology.[37]

Many modern sourdough breads are prepared using faster-acting chemical methods or leavening agents that require only a few hours and do not utilize the extended fermentation of wheat flour by sourdough bacteria. As a result, there is not enough time for the microbes in the dough to process and break down the gluten to low levels, as in traditionally prepared sourdough.

This is another example of how traditional food preparation can have health advantages that are lost when foods are prepared using modern, time-saving methods. To be clear, I'm not recommending that patients with celiac disease or gluten sensitivity consume sourdough bread (or einkorn wheat)—reactions vary, and wheat in any form may not be tolerated. Instead, transitioning from wheat bread to sourdough bread may be a good initial step for people who are trying to reduce the amount of gluten in their diet.

What about if you don't have celiac disease or any known gluten sensitivity? Should you still eliminate gluten? This question must be individualized. One way to test this would be to do an elimination diet. Eliminate gluten for at least three months and then reintroduce it and observe the effects on your body. If you want data to guide you, further testing is possible through functional medicine, a branch of integrative medicine that uses specialized lab testing to assess the function of different organ systems. Several laboratories offer functional medicine tests for gluten sensitivity, utilizing blood, saliva, or stool samples, that go beyond the traditional qualitative blood test for celiac disease by quantifying the degree of gluten sensitivity. Determining which lab and which test is right for you is a clinical decision best made in conjunction with a functional medicine practitioner.

If you have autoimmune disease of any kind, inflammatory bowel disease, or hypothyroidism, it is likely that a gluten-free diet would be beneficial for you. There is evidence also that the gluten-free diet can be helpful for patients with a variety of neurological disorders, including chronic migraine, epilepsy, and Parkinson's disease.[38] In my clinic, I also find that a gluten-free diet is beneficial for patients with imbalances in their gut bacteria, as part of a comprehensive program to optimize and restore the health of their microbiome. To find out more about whether you can eat wheat, take the following quiz.

## Gluten Compatibility Quiz: Can I Eat Wheat?

Answer yes or no to the following statements:

- I have a healthy microbiome, as assessed by a functional medicine practitioner OR I have a score of 9 or higher on the microbiome assessment quiz in Chapter 5.
- I don't have any autoimmune disease, such as celiac disease, Hashimoto's disease, or inflammatory bowel disease.
- I don't have prediabetes or diabetes.
- My fasting insulin level is below 10.
- I don't have irritable bowel syndrome or digestive symptoms such as heartburn, bloating, excessive gas, constipation, or diarrhea.
- I don't have unexplained chronic conditions such as recurrent migraines, chronic fatigue syndrome, ADHD, or anxiety/depression.
- My functional medicine practitioner has ruled out non-celiac gluten sensitivity with specialized lab testing.
- Based on laboratory testing, I don't have any genes that predispose me to celiac disease or gluten sensitivity.
- I have tried eliminating gluten for at least two months before and don't feel noticeably better on a gluten-free diet.
- I'm willing to consume only stone-ground whole wheat berries from organic non-GMO ancient grains (such as einkorn or emmer) that are cooked through traditional means like soaking and/or sprouting followed by long-term fermentation.

*How Did You Do?*

Count up the number of "Yes" answers that you have.

**Score: 10.** I'm comfortable recommending that you try eating properly cooked and prepared ancient grains of wheat and see how you feel. If you tolerate them well, consuming them in moderation should be okay.

**Score: 8-9.** This is a borderline score. Under certain conditions, you may still be able to tolerate properly cooked and prepared wheat. However, there may be significant long-term risks if any of the above criteria are not met.

**Score: 7 or below.** You are probably better off not consuming wheat, because of possible risks in terms of worsening autoimmune disease, harmful metabolic consequences, and/or other adverse effects.

I hope it doesn't seem like this quiz is excessively strict or impractical. These are just all the different factors that are genuinely important to help determine whether you'll be able to tolerate wheat without any adverse health effects. I do have some patients who scored a ten and consume wheat while seeming to maintain good health and overall vitality.

## My Personal Approach to Wheat

In case you're wondering, I score high enough to tolerate wheat but still do not eat it. Why? There are several reasons. One of my goals with my daily diet is to maximize nutrient density. Eating foods such as vegetables and other superfoods (please see Chapter 4 for more details) enables me to get more nutrients into my body than through eating wheat. I think about this as the opportunity cost of food—whatever you eat limits your ability to consume other foods. I also have a family history of diabetes and try to consume a diet with a low glycemic index, so avoiding most grains is helpful with this. I don't have the time or desire to track down organic, non-GMO whole-wheat berries from ancient grains and properly soak and ferment them. I also did not grow up eating a lot of foods containing wheat (rice was our staple), so I don't have a particularly strong desire to consume wheat based on childhood experience.

There is nothing unique to wheat that cannot be obtained from other foods, and there may be potential disadvantages to wheat. For example, it is clear that components of wheat such as gluten are hard to digest and may promote increased intestinal permeability, gut inflammation, and an immune response even in healthy individuals.[39] Also, there is an increasingly understood link between gluten sensitivity and autoimmune disease, one of our epidemic modern diseases.[40]

Many of my patients, for similar reasons, have decided to go gluten-free and avoid eating wheat. For all people, if they've never tried eliminating gluten, I recommend they at least try that once, in a program such as the Paleovedic Detox outlined in Chapter 12. If they've never tried cutting out wheat to see if they feel better, it makes sense to try that at least once to see if it makes a difference for them. In my clinical practice, almost everyone scores 7 or below, so I recommend a gluten-free diet to most of my patients.

With that said, it is possible for certain people who score a 10 on my quiz to eat properly cooked and prepared ancient grains of wheat occasionally as part of a healthy diet. I say occasionally because with all foods it is a good idea to rotate them and not eat the same food every day. Our bodies were designed for variety, and eating the same foods every day can sometimes cause the body to develop immune reactions such as food sensitivities against those foods.

For those who scored a 10 and are interested in exploring heirloom grains and traditional wheat preparation practices, there are a few resources online that could be helpful:

- The Weston Price foundation has a number of articles that are informative: www.westonaprice.org/modern-diseases/against-the-grain/
- This website discusses how to bake traditional sourdough bread using natural cultures and without commercial yeast: www.realsourdoughbreadrecipe.com/
- If you have gluten sensitivity but crave sourdough bread, I recommend this recipe for gluten-free sourdough: www.wholenewmom.com/recipes/gluten-free-sourdough-starter

## Gluten-free Grains

What about other grains besides wheat? Anthropologists have found that a number of grains have been consumed by other traditional populations for between five thousand to ten thousand years; these include rice in Asia, corn in Central and South America, millet and sorghum in Africa, and barley in the Middle East.[41] While it's true that many of these cultures consumed grain since the advent of agriculture about ten thousand years ago, there is still a longer period of about two million years before the advent of agriculture when grains were probably not cultivated consistently.

During this time, hunter-gatherer populations generally consumed meat whenever possible, but wild plants, roots, and tubers would have comprised the main source of their caloric intake. As I mentioned earlier, certain ancestral populations such as the Kitavans in Papua New Guinea consume mostly carbohydrates and almost no animal protein. As agriculture has taken hold over the past ten thousand years, there have been certain changes in our DNA that have started to adapt us to incorporating grains into our diet.

For example, the genes that encode starch digestion may be multiplied in populations that consume larger amounts of starch. There are significant differences between individuals in the activity of a salivary enzyme called amylase that starts to break down starch; these differences may make certain people better able to digest and break down starch without adverse insulin responses.[42] The gene that encodes the salivary enzyme amylase is AMY1. Studies have shown that some people have more copies of this gene, enabling them to produce significantly more amylase and thereby more efficiently digest starches; it seems that, over time, populations that practice farming have gradually gained more copies of the AMY1 gene, while nonfarming populations have had a relatively stable number of AMY1 copies.[43]

While these initial changes are interesting, they definitely do not make us "adapted" to thrive on refined grains or other components of the Western diets such as vegetable oils and excess sugar. The vast majority of our genetic code is still shaped by the 2.5 million years we lived as hunter-gatherers before the advent of agriculture.

## Healthy Starches for All

Healthy starches are an important part of the Paleovedic Diet program. Healthy starches that almost all people can tolerate are starchy tubers. These include potatoes, beets, sweet potatoes, squash, yams, yucca, cassava, or taro root. It's well established that many traditional populations (and human ancestors) consumed starchy vegetables. Of note, many of these foods are FODMAPs and contain components that are fermented by your gut bacteria. If you have any imbalances in your microbiome, such as small intestinal bacterial overgrowth

(SIBO) or irritable bowel syndrome, these foods could sometimes make your symptoms worse. Going on a low-FODMAP diet while you work on rebalancing your microbiome can be a good therapeutic intervention. However, this should be only for a limited time while you are working on your gut under the supervision of your functional medicine practitioner. Permanently reducing or eliminating these foods is not a good idea, because you are taking away from the diet all the foods that can potentially strengthen and support your beneficial bacteria.

Experiment with different starches to see what works best for you. Focusing on complex carbohydrates with a lower glycemic load and lower carbohydrate density can help ensure that you are getting the optimal carbs in your diet and all the benefits that carbohydrates can bring. Above all, don't be afraid of carbs.

# CHAPTER 3
# ALL ABOUT FATS AND PROTEIN

In this chapter, we focus on the other two important categories of macronutrients: fats and protein. Let me begin by stating that fat is not the enemy. In fact, scientists believe that increasing rates of obesity are related more to excess carbohydrate and sugar consumption than to fat intake. The widely prevalent myth that dietary fat causes heart disease has been debunked. Unfortunately, based on public health advice to reduce fat intake, food manufacturers have often replaced fat in food with sugar—part of the reason we as a society are overweight.

## Good Fats vs. Bad Fats

It is quite clear now what fats are beneficial and what fats are harmful. Good fats include extra-virgin olive oil, avocados, oil from fish, butter from grass-fed cows, ghee (clarified butter), fermented full-fat dairy, pasteurized eggs, coconut oil, unheated nut oils, nuts, seeds, and grass-fed meats. Harmful fats include trans fats, hydrogenated fats, and vegetable seed oils. Vegetable oils that I recommend avoiding because of high omega-6 content, genetic modification, and excessive industrial processing include peanut oil, canola oil, soybean oil, corn oil, cottonseed oil, safflower oil, grapeseed oil, and sunflower oil.

Fatty acids can be classified as saturated, monounsaturated, or polyunsaturated, depending on their chemical structure. The good fats listed above come from all three categories. Saturated fats are solid at room temperature, while polyunsaturated fats are liquid.

## Is Saturated Fat Harmful?

The type of fat that doctors have been vehemently warning people about for years is saturated fat, and yet research shows that saturated fat is not the villain it has been made out to be. A large meta-analysis reviewing studies including 350,000 people concluded that there is no evidence that consuming saturated fat is associated with increased risk of heart disease or stroke.[1] Another systematic review evaluating studies with over 600,000 people found that there is no evidence to support the recommendation to reduce saturated fat intake and increase polyunsaturated fat consumption in order to prevent cardiovascular disease.[2] Therefore, saturated fats are safe to consume as part of a well-balanced diet.

## Coconut Oil

One of the healthiest fats, coconut oil, actually consists of 91 percent saturated fat. Interestingly, certain Polynesian populations consume up to 60 percent of their calories from coconut (thus getting more than 50 percent of calories from fat) and appear to be quite healthy, without any sign of cardiovascular disease.[3]

Most of the fatty acids in coconut oil are medium chain triglycerides (MCTs), which have unique health benefits. MCTs help to reduce hunger and boost metabolism and baseline energy expenditure. One double-blind study found that a small daily intake of dietary MCT was able to boost resting energy expenditure by 5 percent, equivalent to about 120 calories per day.[4] This is one way that coconut oil can promote weight loss, in addition to its effect on reducing appetite.

Coconut oil seems especially helpful at reducing abdominal fat and favorably affecting cholesterol. In one study, women who were given two tablespoons of coconut oil per day had significant reduction in belly fat and a beneficial increase in HDL cholesterol after twelve weeks.[5]

Finally, coconut oil is a natural antimicrobial, helping to inhibit the growth of harmful bacteria, viruses, and fungi. I sometimes use a coconut oil-derived compound called monolaurin to help treat pathogenic bacterial overgrowth in the gut. Coconut oil is a pillar of the Paleovedic Diet because of its extraordinary health benefits.

## Monounsaturated Fats

Almost everyone agrees that monounsaturated fats, such as olive oil and avocados, are healthy. Most nuts and seeds are also rich sources of monounsaturated fats. Interestingly, the much-maligned fat lard is about 40 percent monounsaturated fat (with the rest being mostly saturated fat), making it a fairly innocuous option nutritionally. It is stable at high temperatures and therefore a good option for cooking, like clarified butter or ghee. Be sure to get lard from pasture-raised animals, as lard from conventional meat can be too high in omega-6 fats.

## Polyunsaturated Fats: Omega-3 vs. Omega-6

There are two main types of polyunsaturated fats: omega-3 and omega-6. Historically, the optimal ratio of omega-6 to omega-3 fats in the body was 1:1. Now many people have up to a 20:1 ratio, which promotes inflammation and cellular damage and can lead to a variety of health problems.

Some health professionals still group all polyunsaturated fats into the same category despite the strong evidence that omega-6 fats have very different effects in the body than omega-3 fats. A number of studies have looked at this issue. One observational study found that as the ratio between omega-3 and omega-6 increased (with more omega-3 and less omega-6), the inflammatory marker C-reactive protein (CRP) decreased proportionally.[6] Higher intake of omega-3 fatty acids has been linked to lower levels of inflammatory markers such as CRP and other blood tests.[7]

This holds true in healthy people and has been demonstrated in patient populations with coronary artery disease[8] and breast cancer.[9] Conversely, elevated levels of omega-6 have been linked to increased inflammation, and recommendations for substituting saturated fat with polyunsaturated fat without differentiating between omega-6 and omega-3 could potentially increase a person's risk of heart disease.

What does all this mean for you? The best approach is to simultaneously focus on both increasing omega-3 and reducing omega-6 in the diet. I would suggest aiming for a ratio of between 4:1 and 5:1. The following tables can provide helpful guidance as you strive to increase the omega-3s and reduce the omega-6s in your diet.

## Omega-3 and Omega-6 Content in Foods

The following charts illustrate the omega-3 and omega-6 content of different categories of foods. For each category, the foods are listed in ascending order (lowest to highest) of omega-6 content. Limiting total intake of omega-6 fatty acids and increasing omega-3 consumption is beneficial; the following tables will help guide you in achieving this. Remember that you want to aim for a ratio of omega-6 to omega-3 fats in your diet of 4:1. For example, if you get 2,500 mg per day of omega-3 fats through fish or seafood consumption, in order to maintain the 4:1 ratio, you would need to consume no more than 10,000 mg or 10 g of omega-6 fats each day. As you can see from the data in the tables, without some attention to detail, you might easily go over this amount and end up consuming more omega-6 fats than is optimal. For example, three handfuls of almonds would already give you more than 10 g of omega-6 fats.

Also remember that fish and seafood have long-chain omega-3 fatty acids such as EPA and DHA, which are more beneficial and health-promoting than the short-chain omega-3 fats such as ALA in nuts, seeds, and plant oils. ALA can be converted to EPA and DHA in the body, but this conversion is less than 10 percent in most people.

## OMEGA-3 vs. OMEGA-6 IN PLANT FATS AND OILS

| Plant Fats and Oils, per 100 grams (3.5 oz) | Omega-6 mg (lowest to highest) | Omega-3 (ALA) mg |
|---|---|---|
| Coconut oil | 1,800 | 0 |
| Macadamia nut oil | 2,400 | 0 |
| Palm oil* | 9,100 | 200 |
| Olive oil | 9,763 | 761 |
| Hazelnut oil | 10,101 | 0 |
| Avocado oil | 12,531 | 957 |
| Flaxseed oil | 12,701 | 53,300 |
| Canola, high oleic | 14,503 | 9,137 |
| Safflower oil, high oleic | 14,350 | 0 |
| Mustard oil | 15,332 | 5,900 |
| Almond oil | 17,401 | 0 |
| Peanut oil | 31,711 | 0 |
| Rice bran oil | 33,402 | 1,600 |
| Sesame oil | 41,304 | 300 |

| Plant Fats and Oils, per 100 grams (3.5 oz) | Omega-6 mg (lowest to highest) | Omega-3 (ALA) mg |
|---|---|---|
| Soybean oil | 50,293 | 7,033 |
| Cottonseed oil | 51,503 | 200 |
| Walnut oil | 52,894 | 10,401 |
| Corn oil | 53,510 | 1,161 |
| Sunflower oil (linoleic) | 65,702 | 0 |
| Grapeseed oil | 69,591 | 100 |
| Safflower oil (linoleic) | 74,615 | 0 |

*Palm oil is not generally recommended due to sustainability concerns (refer to page 47 for details).

You may wonder exactly how much is 100 g of oil? While it varies depending on the specific oil, 100 g of oil is generally equivalent to about 7 tablespoons, or a little less than half a cup.

## OMEGA-3 vs. OMEGA-6 IN ANIMAL FATS

| Animal Fats, per 100 g | Omega-6 mg per 100 g | Omega-3 mg |
|---|---|---|
| Butter oil | 2,247 | 1,417 |
| Butter | 2,728 | 315 |
| Ghee (clarified butter) | 2,728 | 315 |
| Beef tallow | 3,100 | 600 |
| Lard (from pork) | 10,199 | 1,000 |
| Duck fat | 11,999 | 1,000 |
| Chicken fat | 19,503 | 1,000 |
| Turkey fat | 21,201 | 1,400 |

# OMEGA-3 vs. OMEGA-6 IN MEAT

| Meat, per 100 g | Omega-6 (approximate) | Omega-3 (approximate) |
|---|---|---|
| Beef, grass-fed, lean | 90 | 23 |
| Goat | 100 | 20 |
| Lamb, lean | 150–300 | 100–200 |
| Venison | 220 | 100 |
| Bison | 200–300 | 80 |
| Beef, grain-fed, lean | 300 | 10–30 |
| Pork, lean | 300 | 10 |
| Ostrich | 350 | 70 |
| Rabbit | 360 | 140 |
| Beef, grass-fed, not lean | 420 | 86 |
| Chicken liver | 400–700 | 140–290 |
| Duck breast, wild | 510 | 10 |
| Turkey, light meat | 550 | 20–60 |
| Chicken, light meat | 690 | 76 |
| Chicken, thigh meat | 1,890 | 120–150 |
| Eggs, whole scrambled | 1,916 | 154 |
| Turkey, meat and skin | 2,940 | 280 |
| Chicken, dark meat and skin | 3,040 | 190–240 |
| Duck, meat and skin | 3,360 | 60 |
| Eggs, yolks only | 3,538 | 282 |
| Bacon | 5,020 | 480 |

How large is a portion of 100 g of meat? While it varies based on the type of meat, 100 g is equivalent to 3.5 ounces, which is about the size of a deck of cards or a computer mouse.

## OMEGA-3 vs. OMEGA-6 IN NUTS AND SEEDS

| Nuts and seeds per 100 g | Omega-6 | Omega-3 (short-chain ALA) |
|---|---|---|
| Coconut, dried | 706 | 0 |
| Macadamia | 1,296 | 206 |
| Hazelnut (filbert) | 5,499 | 87 |
| Chia seed | 5,785 | 17,552 |
| Flaxseed | 5,911 | 22,813 |
| Cashew | 7,782 | 161 |
| Almond | 12,053 | 6 |
| Pistachio | 13,636 | 254 |
| Brazil nut | 20,564 | 18 |
| Pecan | 20,630 | 986 |
| Pumpkin seed | 20,703 | 166 |
| Sesame seed | 25,226 | 376 |
| Pine nut | 33,606 | 112 |
| Sunflower seed | 37,389 | 79 |
| Walnut | 38,092 | 9,079 |

How much is 100 g of nuts? This is equivalent to 3.5 ounces, which is about 3 handfuls of nuts (1 handful of nuts is approximately 1 ounce).

## OMEGA-3 vs. OMEGA-6 IN SEAFOOD

With this table, the foods have been arranged in descending order of omega-3 content starting with the foods with the highest omega-3 levels. These are the types of seafood that you should generally try to eat more of.

| Fish and Seafood, per 100 g | Omega-6 | Omega-3 (long-chain EPA and DHA) |
|---|---|---|
| Fish caviar, black or red | 81 | 6,789 |
| Mackerel, Atlantic | 219 | 2,670 |
| Salmon, Atlantic, wild | 172 | 2,586 |
| Salmon, Atlantic, farmed | 982 | 2,506 |
| Herring, Pacific | 192 | 2,418 |
| Salmon, Chinook | 472 | 2,418 |
| Tuna, blue fin | 68 | 1,664 |
| Mackerel, Pacific | 116 | 1,614 |
| Sardine, Atlantic | 110 | 1,480 |
| Salmon, sockeye, canned | 152 | 1,323 |
| Trout | 224 | 1,068 |
| Bluefish | 60 | 1,067 |
| Swordfish | 30 | 825 |
| Oysters, Pacific | 32 | 740 |
| Halibut | 38 | 669 |
| Eel | 196 | 653 |
| Shrimp, canned | 28 | 601 |
| Flatfish (flounder, sole) | 8 | 563 |
| Lobster | 13 | 534 |
| Mussels, blue | 18 | 482 |
| Clams | 32 | 396 |
| Scallop | 4 | 396 |
| Crab | 8 | 382 |
| Snapper | 25 | 343 |

| Fish and Seafood, per 100 g | Omega-6 | Omega-3 (long-chain EPA and DHA) |
|---|---|---|
| Octopus | 9 | 326 |
| Tuna, yellow fin | 10 | 243 |
| Tilapia | 300 | 240 |
| Cod, Pacific | 8 | 221 |
| Crayfish | 76 | 184 |

Tables adapted with permission from Julianne Taylor, paleozonenutrition.com

## Fish—The Ultimate Healthy Fat

It is clear that fish consumption is one of the best things you can do for your health. Studies show that eating fish is beneficial for reducing the risk of heart disease. One recent meta-analysis that included over 400,000 people concluded that fish consumption appears significantly beneficial in the prevention of heart attacks, and higher consumption was associated with correspondingly greater protection.[10] Interestingly, the benefit seems greater for consumption of whole fish rather than consumption of fish oil supplements. Eating a whole food seems more beneficial than taking supplements with isolated components of food. Consumption of fish seems to be more effective at raising the intracellular levels of omega-3s than taking fish oil supplements.[11]

With fish there are legitimate concerns about mercury, dioxins, PCBs, and other toxins. I don't believe that the presence of these toxins outweighs the remarkable health benefits of consuming good-quality fish. I recommend consuming seafood that is known to be lower in mercury. The smaller the fish, the less likely it is to have significant amounts of toxins, which tend to accumulate in larger fish higher in the food chain. The Monterey Bay Aquarium and the Environmental Working Group websites provide guidance on which fish are environmentally sustainable and low in toxins. Because of the outstanding omega-3 content of fish, I recommend trying to aim for at least half a pound of cold-water fish each week. Good options are salmon, sardines, herring, anchovies, and mackerel.

## Palm Oil

Palm oil, especially unrefined red palm oil, consists mostly of saturated and monounsaturated fats, making it a fairly good option nutritionally; it is sought out by food manufacturers trying to replace trans fats in their products. Palm oil is extracted from the fruit of the palm tree, while palm kernel oil is extracted from the seed of the fruit. Red palm oil is a good source of vitamin E as well. However, there are significant social and environmental concerns about the production of palm oil, including issues of deforestation and its consequences, such as habitat destruction of endangered species.[12] Unless such concerns about sustainability are specifically addressed, palm oil is not recommended—certain brands now offer fairly traded, certified organic, sustainably sourced red palm oil.

## Ghee

Ghee is often used for therapeutic purposes in Ayurveda. It is considered to be a brain tonic and to be helpful for stimulating the digestive fire and building ojas, which corresponds to vitality. It is used as an aid to detoxification in Ayurveda. It can also be used as a delivery vehicle for various herbs because it helps increase the potency of herbs.

### Make Your Own Ghee

While ghee is available commercially, it can be expensive, and making your own ghee is relatively easy and fun. To begin, purchase a good quality, organic grass–fed butter. You can use either salted or unsalted butter, but I prefer salted butter because unsalted butter can have other ingredients like lactic acid instead of salt.

Take 4 4-ounce quarters (total of 16 ounces) of the butter and melt them in a pan uncovered at medium heat. When the butter is fully melted, turn the stove to the lowest possible heat and let the butter simmer. Stir occasionally for the first 5 minutes and continue to simmer for about 30 to 40 minutes. The butter will make a bubbling, crackling noise, and some foam will appear on the top.

As it is cooking, particles from the butter will sink to the bottom and form a brownish solid residue. A fragrant smell like freshly made popcorn will fill your kitchen. After 30 to 40 minutes, when the butter has stopped crackling and bubbling, check to see if the ghee is done—put a drop of water into the ghee. If it's done, the ghee will crackle briefly as the water evaporates and then stop crackling. Now the ghee is ready. Skim off the foam and discard it. Pour the clear liquid through a strainer into a glass jar and allow it to cool before closing the lid. Ghee has a very long shelf life and should not be refrigerated.

## Full-fat Dairy Protects against Diabetes

If you tolerate them, full-fat dairy products can be a healthy part of your diet. Milk consumption is often limited because of widespread lactose intolerance. As we get older, most of us lose the enzymes necessary to digest the lactose in milk. Other milk products, such as butter, ghee, cheese, kefir, and yogurt, are relatively low in lactose and better tolerated. Grass-fed butter is rich in vitamin A, vitamin D, conjugated linolenic acid (CLA), omega-3 fatty acids, and vitamin $K_2$ (an important nutrient for bone health that is found only in dairy products and a few other foods). Fermented dairy such as yogurt and kefir is especially rich in probiotics.

In addition, research shows that consumption of full-fat dairy products is associated with a decreased risk of developing diabetes—one study followed twenty-seven thousand people over around fourteen years and found that people who consumed eight portions of full-fat dairy per day (cream, cheese, milk, or yogurt) had a 23 percent lower chance of developing diabetes than people who consumed one or fewer portions of full-fat dairy per day.[13] There was no benefit for people who consumed low-fat dairy. The study was consistent with earlier studies that demonstrated that dairy product consumption could protect against the development of insulin resistance and diabetes.[14,15]

What could be the mechanism behind this benefit? One potential ingredient is trans-palmitoleic acid, a fatty acid that is found in full-fat dairy products. One study found that higher circulating levels of trans-palmitoleic acid were associated with higher HDL levels, lower triglyceride levels, less insulin resistance, and a reduced incidence of diabetes.[16] However, dairy products are complex whole foods that contain a variety of nutrients, and it is hard to attribute their benefit to just one component.

## Low-fat Dairy Can Be Harmful to Health

If you tolerate dairy and consume it, I recommend having full-fat dairy. This is because full-fat dairy is a whole food and must be processed significantly in order to remove part or all of the fat content. Food processing has unpredictable effects that can sometimes be harmful to health.

For example, one study from the Harvard School of Public Health of eighteen thousand women found that low-fat dairy products can potentially reduce fertility.[17] One of the common causes of infertility in women is anovulation, where the woman fails to ovulate or release an egg into the fallopian tubes during her monthly cycle. Low-fat dairy products were found to be associated with a higher incidence of anovulatory infertility, while full-fat dairy products were in fact associated with a reduced incidence of anovulation. The authors of the study recommend that women trying to conceive substitute full-fat dairy products for low-fat dairy products.[18] My philosophy is that eating whole foods is superior to eating processed foods, and the research confirms this in the area of dairy products.

## The Importance of Protein

Proteins are the basic building blocks of life. The importance of protein for growth and development are well known, especially since the structure and function of nearly every organ and tissue depend on protein. Perhaps less well-known are the roles of protein in blood sugar balance, immune system function, hormone synthesis, and the activity of enzymes and neurotransmitters. In fact, protein plays a role in almost every physiological process. Therefore, getting adequate protein is essential.

## How Much Protein Should I Eat?

Government guidelines recommend consuming about 0.36 g of protein per pound of body weight—for example, 54 g of protein per day for a 150-pound person. I have heard some holistic practitioners recommend up to 0.8 g of protein per pound of body weight per day, which is the upper end of the spectrum. Most people get between 15 and 20 percent of calories from protein.

Protein requirements vary widely based on activity level, body weight goals, and overall health, and there are times when a higher percentage could be helpful. For example, increasing protein intake can help promote weight loss, build muscle mass, stabilize blood sugar, or recover from chronic illness. Studies show that the increased feeling of fullness that protein provides can significantly help facilitate weight loss; therefore, if you are trying lose weight, eating more protein can be beneficial.[19] Those trying to build muscle or better handle blood sugar issues would also benefit from increased protein intake.

There is an important difference based on your Ayurvedic body type. Vata types need the most protein and should generally consume protein with every meal. Kapha types need the least amount of protein, and pitta types have a moderate need. Consider your Ayurvedic type, your body weight goals, and your individual circumstances when determining how much protein you need every day.

## Should I Eat Meat?

Can one be healthy while following a vegetarian or vegan diet? There is a lot of dogma and strong opinions on this subject in various books on ancestral diets. For example, from *Paleoista*, by Nell Stephenson, "Humans simply cannot get enough protein if they do not eat flesh. Period." On the other extreme are authors such as Dr. John McDougall. In his recent book, *The Starch Solution,* he describes an ideal diet as "one that reduces or eliminates animal foods such as meat, dairy, and eggs."[20] According to Ayurveda, the answer lies somewhere in the middle and depends on your body type, as we will discuss later.

Ayurveda explains why certain people might do well on a vegetarian diet, while others may do better while consuming animal protein. Historical factors such as the type of diet that populations evolved to eat over time affect their genetics and their adaptation to different diets. For example, certain populations in India have followed a vegetarian diet over thousands of years and in fact are well-adapted to maintain health without eating meat.

In contrast, the Masai people of Africa subsist mainly on meat, milk, and blood from animals. Genetic analysis has identified certain factors that enable them to be healthy and adapt to consuming almost 100 percent of their calories from animal foods.

## Health Concerns about Eating Meat

Let's look at some of the common health objections to eating meat.[21]

1. It is high in cholesterol.

Cholesterol used to be vilified because of the suspected connection to heart disease. We now know that heart disease is more related to inflammation and not directly caused by elevated cholesterol. Moreover, cholesterol is an essential nutrient that is part of the cell membrane of every cell in your body. Most of your cholesterol is made in your liver every day. In fact, studies show that in about 75 percent of people, changing dietary cholesterol has no significant effect on blood cholesterol levels, and for the remaining 25 percent, reduction of dietary cholesterol has only a minor effect on serum cholesterol.[22]

2. It is high in saturated fat.

Saturated fat is another dietary component that has been falsely blamed for the putative link to heart disease. As I discussed above, research reveals that saturated fat in moderation is not harmful and is not associated with increased risk of disease.

3. It is high in protein, and Americans consume too much protein.

This may be partially true in that Americans often do consume more protein than they need. However, excess protein from any source—plant or animal—can be harmful. In fact, many plant foods can be very high in protein as well. While it is true that excess protein does have a potentially harmful effect on the body and on kidney function, it does not mean that avoiding meat is necessary in order to prevent excessive consumption of protein. What is needed is tracking one's overall protein intake and ensuring that is not excessive.

4. It is high in methionine.

Methionine is a sulfur-containing amino acid that is present in animal foods. This statement is true insofar as the types of meat that are consumed in the

United States, mainly muscle meats, are high in methionine. However, eating nose-to-tail, which involves eating organ meats and all parts of the animal, balances the amino acids that are consumed. Some state that methionine is metabolized into homocysteine in the body, which is a potential risk factor for cardiovascular disease and other chronic diseases. However, in my experience, homocysteine levels are more affected by problems with breaking down homocysteine normally rather than excessive consumption of dietary methionine. Homocysteine breakdown is affected by methylation pathways and genetic mutations, as well as B-vitamin deficiencies. Addressing these is more important for managing homocysteine than regulating dietary methionine levels.

5. It is high in dietary acids.

Certain diet programs emphasize avoiding animal foods because they are high in acids. The theory is that these acids stimulate bones to release calcium and other alkaline materials to neutralize them, thereby promoting osteoporosis. While there was some initial research supporting this idea,[23] the latest articles by the same researchers refute the idea that animal foods in some way leach minerals such as calcium from your bones. Dr. Thomas Remer, a prolific researcher in this field, recently wrote, "Although in the past high protein intake was often assumed to exert a primarily detrimental impact on bone mass and skeletal health, the majority of recent studies indicates the opposite and suggests a bone-anabolic (bone-building) influence."[24]

One study cited to support this idea looked at patients who consumed excessive animal protein *and did not eat fruits and vegetables*; this study acknowledged that when patients eat enough fruits and vegetables, there is no harmful effect on bone loss from meat.[25] Researchers in another study reiterated that it's more important to focus on consuming adequate fruits and vegetables than reducing dietary protein: "concerns about the impact of protein on acid production appear to be minor compared with the alkalinizing effects of fruits and vegetables."[26]

6. It is a nutritionally poor choice.

Meat is a nutrient-dense food that is rich in protein, vitamins, minerals, and healthy fats. It is true that there is a significant nutritional difference between commercial feedlot-raised meat and organic or grass-fed meat. For example, grass-fed beef is significantly higher in omega-3 fatty acids than commercial grain-fed beef. In addition, organ meats such as liver are among the most nutrient-dense foods on the planet, with highly bioavailable forms of vitamin A, B vitamins, and minerals.

7. Red meat is especially bad for you.

Red meat is often believed to be disease promoting. However, there is a big difference between unprocessed red meat and meat that has been processed with preservatives, nitrates, and other chemicals—these include deli meats, luncheon meats, hot dogs, and so forth. One large meta-analysis that included over 1.2 million people in twenty studies concluded that unprocessed red meat was not associated with increased risk of heart disease, diabetes, or stroke, whereas processed red meat was associated with higher risk of heart disease and diabetes.[27] Other studies have also found differences based on whether or not meat is processed. Also, charring or broiling meat at high temperatures produces potentially carcinogenic compounds such as heterocyclic amines (HCAs) and polycyclic aromatic hydrocarbons (PAHs) and should be avoided.

Therefore, unprocessed grass-fed red meats cooked at low temperatures are acceptable in moderation and do not carry health risks as part of a balanced diet.

## Environmental and Moral Issues with Meat

During my years as a vegetarian, I became intimately aware of the environmental and ethical arguments against eating meat. Most vegetarians are aware that producing one pound of animal protein requires far more natural resources such as water and air than producing one pound of vegetables. These are very real issues given the environmental and population issues that we are faced with. I am still acutely aware of these issues and do my best to purchase meat and fish that is organic, pasture-raised and finished, and environmentally sustainable. Plant foods should comprise the majority of the diet for all people.

In terms of the ethical arguments, a lot could be written about the moral and ethical implications of eating meat. For ethical reasons, I decided to become vegetarian when I was younger and subsequently struggled with the ethical ramifications when I eventually returned to eating meat several years later. In this book, I am not trying to take a moral stance on this issue. My advice is morally neutral and focused only on the health implications.

## Can I Be a Healthy Vegetarian?

Ayurveda believes that the answer is yes, but there are a few factors to consider. First, it depends on your body type. Vata constitutional types may have the hardest time being vegetarian. They require significantly higher protein intake, and the heavy, grounding properties of meat are especially beneficial for them. As a vata type myself, I definitely struggled with my health during the years I was a vegetarian. In contrast, pitta and kapha types have relatively lower requirements for protein, and kapha types may be considered to be best-suited for vegetarianism. In fact, kapha types can even theoretically do well on a vegan diet (with the appropriate supplements)—I have a number of kapha patients who are healthy vegans. It is well known that vegetarians are at increased risk for certain deficiencies, such as of vitamin $B_{12}$, zinc, magnesium, and essential fatty acids, so being vegetarian does require more effort to pay attention to these potential pitfalls.

Ayurveda also believes that you should take into account what your ancestors ate and that populations can adapt to being vegetarian over time. In India, the caste system, which facilitated a division of labor and social organization, also provided guidelines about diet. For example, the Brahmin or priestly class was strictly vegetarian. Some people can trace their genealogy for dozens of generations through their caste. It is possible that being Brahmin over thousands of years could lead to genetic changes that would enable one to be healthy while adhering to a vegetarian diet. I know many people from this caste who are thriving on a vegetarian diet. In contrast, I come from the Kshatriya or warrior caste, which traditionally always eats meat. Ayurveda would consider this an important factor in determining my diet today.

Of course, for the great majority of human evolution, all people were hunter-gatherers and subsisted on starchy tubers, vegetables, fruits, and most likely meat when available. However, Ayurveda believes that over time populations can adapt to different diets—we saw evidence of this in the increases in salivary enzyme levels in farming populations that we discussed earlier. Therefore, it can be helpful to look at the short-term dietary patterns of your ancestors in the previous hundreds of years as well. Do some research into the traditional diets of your distant ancestors, and see what lessons you can learn from them.

Finally, Ayurveda believes that the ultimate test of any diet is experience. Try being vegetarian for a while, and see how you feel, especially in terms of energy levels, mood, digestion, and vitality. This was a test that I failed, as my health gradually deteriorated when I was vegetarian, despite the fact that I ate lots of protein and took appropriate supplements. If you feel fantastic on a vegetarian diet, by all means continue that and be sure to supplement wisely to continue maintaining good health.

## Choosing the Best Quality Meats—How to Read Labels

If you do decide to eat meat, it can be confusing to differentiate between all the different package labels out there—organic, free-range, pasture-raised, grass-fed, and others. There is a noticeable difference between pasture-raised natural meat and its factory-farmed counterpart, both in terms of taste and nutritional value. Unfortunately, the term "natural" on packaged meats is misleading because there is no industry-wide standard for what "natural" means, and as a result this term is meaningless.

Let's review some examples of what different terms might mean, taking beef and chicken as an example.

### Beef

- **Pastured or grass-fed and finished**—this means that the animal was raised on pasture and was fed grass throughout its life. This is the healthiest option.
- **Grass-fed and grain-finished**—often, grass-fed beef is fed grass for most of its life and then is given grain for additional weight gain for a period of time. Such beef is certainly preferable to conventional grain-fed beef but not as good as beef that has been fed only grass (grass-fed and finished).
- **Organic**—technically, beef that is fed organic grains can be certified organic. If it does not specifically say that it is grass-fed, there is no way to know what type of feed the animal was given. Therefore, the term *organic* is actually somewhat less important than grass-fed when it comes to beef.
- **Conventional**—comes from commercially grain-fed cattle that are often raised in large industrial feedlots. This is the least healthy option.

### Poultry

- **Pastured or pasture-raised**—this means that the birds were raised outdoors with access to foods that are part of their natural diet, such as worms, insects, and so forth. This would be the ideal in terms of meat quality.
- **Organic free-range**—this means that the chickens were raised in a large barn-type structure with access to the outdoors. Unfortunately, this might mean a very small yard, to which the animals rarely venture out. While the chickens are fed organic feed, there are few if any additional positive elements required by this designation.
- **Organic**—this means that the chickens were given organic feed but did not have access to the small outdoor enclosure that "free-range" chickens do (but rarely take advantage of). Therefore, there is not a significant difference between organic and organic free-range.
- **All Natural**—unfortunately, this term does not tell you much at all about the way the animal was raised. You may also see package claims such as hormone-free. However, this is meaningless because federal regulations prohibit the use of hormones in poultry. If it says "Raised without Antibiotics," that is a positive thing because commercial poultry growers do have a choice about this.

### Eggs

- **Pastured**—this means that the eggs were laid by hens out on pasture living in their natural environment. This is the healthiest option.
- **Organic**—this means that the hens were fed certified organic feed and had some outdoor access, but there is no requirement specifying the details of such access.
- **Cage-free**—this means that the birds were typically housed uncaged inside barns but does not specify any requirements for their feed.
- **Farm Fresh or All Natural**—this does not tell you much.

You can see how the terms can get confusing quite easily. The best option is pastured or pasture-raised meat, eggs, and poultry. One could argue that these items are very expensive, but that's where we can show our power as consumers. Our choices have the ability to shift the food industry.

For example, ten years ago there were very few gluten-free products in the market. Now the gluten-free industry is a multibillion dollar business that is rapidly growing and making healthier options available to more people. Unfortunately, gluten-free products are often laden with salt, sugar, or fat, so there's still a long way to go there, but it's evidence of the power of our food choices as consumers.

You may have the good fortune of being able to buy pasture-raised meat directly from farmers, often in larger discounted portions. Our household does not consume enough meat to be able to use these large portions, but we do try to purchase high-quality pastured meats through local natural grocers or online sites such as Tendergrass Farms or US Wellness Meats.

Whether or not you decide to eat meat is a very individual decision. As discussed above, be sure to take into account your Ayurvedic body type, your genetic history, and most importantly the way you feel when you eliminate animal protein from your diet.

# CHAPTER 4

# THE UNKNOWN SUPERFOODS—MAXIMIZING NUTRIENT DENSITY

Americans specialize in eating foods with the lowest numbers of nutrients. I'm not even talking about processed foods or junk food. Americans have an uncanny ability, even among the fresh fruits and vegetables we consume, to choose the least nutritious options. In fact, the most popular fruits and vegetables in America, such as iceberg lettuce (33 pounds per person per year),[1] white potatoes (142 pounds per person per year),[2] corn (56 pounds per person per year),[3] and pears are the most nutrient-poor choices in their respective categories. Moreover, certain popular fruits and vegetables, as we will get to shortly, can even be harmful to health!

By nutrients, I am referring not just to vitamins and minerals but, more importantly, to the health-promoting compounds in plants known as phytochemicals. We used to believe that the benefits of fruits and vegetables derived from vitamins, minerals, and fiber. That has been the basis for traditional rankings of the most nutritious fruits and vegetables. We now know that plants contain hundreds and often thousands of phytochemicals. For example, garlic alone contains over a hundred distinct phytochemicals, which, to me, engenders a sense of awe and respect for the complexity of whole foods. In fact, researchers estimate that up to forty thousand different phytochemicals may be cataloged eventually. We are just beginning to understand all the health benefits of these phytochemicals, which may exceed the benefits of the vitamins and minerals that plants contain.

The major classes of phytonutrients include the following:[4]

- *Organosulfurs*: Examples include the glucosinolates and indoles found in crucifers such as cauliflower and broccoli and the sulfur compounds in garlic.
- *Terpenoids*: These include limonene, which is found in the peels of citrus fruits, as well as carotenoids, coenzyme Q10, phytosterols, tocopherols, and tocotrienols. It also includes xanthophylls like lutein, and zeaxanthin, found in kale.
- *Flavonoids*: Flavonoids are the plant pigments that give plants their colors, like the blue of blueberries (anthocyanidins), the purple of

grapes (resveratrol), or the red of tomatoes (lycopene). Flavonoids also include quercetin, which is found in onions, apples, and citrus fruits, and catechins, present in green tea.

- *Phenolic acids*: Examples include ellagic acids in pomegranates and blackberries, gallic acids from mangoes and strawberries, and hydroxy-cinnamic acids found in blueberries, kiwis, plums, and cherries.
- *Isoflavonoids* and *lignans*: Examples include genistein and diadzein found in soy foods, and the lignans in flaxseed.
- *Aromatic acids*: Ferulic acid, found in oats, oranges, and pineapples, and coumarins, which are found in cinnamon, parsley, and citrus fruits, are examples of aromatic acids.
- *Betalains*: Betanin, betanidin, and betacyanin are part of this new category of antioxidants that are found almost exclusively in red beets.[5]

You might have also heard the term polyphenols, which is a broader category of antioxidants that includes flavonoids, phenolic acids, isoflavonoids, lignans, and aromatic acids. As you can see, there are a large number of phytochemicals, and our understanding of their benefits is growing. The basis for the well-known dietary recommendation to "eat the rainbow" and consume fruits and vegetables of all parts of the color spectrum is to obtain as many different types of phytochemicals as possible, because each color is associated with a different group of nutrients.

Here are some examples of how phytochemicals from fruits and vegetables might protect against one of our modern afflictions, cancer[6]:

- They protect cells from DNA damage, one of the first steps in cancer development.
- They help inactivate carcinogens, which are cancer-promoting chemicals.
- They have antibacterial and antiviral effects, and we know that microbial infection plays a role in certain cancers.
- They have anti-inflammatory effects.
- They inhibit angiogenesis, the mechanism by which tumors grow new blood vessels to sustain themselves.

We learned in Chapter 1 about how a hallmark of blue zone populations is consumption of unprocessed, nutrient-dense foods. Our Paleolithic ancestors also consumed wild fruits and vegetables and benefited from the remarkable diversity and density of nutrients that they contained. In addition, they ate what was fresh and locally available during that season. For example, fruit was not available abundantly year-round but only present for a limited time during particular seasons.

The nutrients in fruits and vegetables comprise one of our primary defenses against disease. However, today's fruits and vegetables are calorie-dense but nutrient-poor—they have limited disease-fighting capacity. This calorie density and nutrient paucity is unfortunately common to both our modern-day fruits and vegetables and packaged or processed foods.

In this chapter (which includes content adapted with permission from Jo Robinson's *Eating on the Wild Side*[7]), we discuss the specific fruits and vegetables that have the highest nutrient density—the unknown and unheralded superfoods—and you will be very surprised by what is on this list and what is not on this list.

In fact, our modern fruits and vegetables were originally derived from wild ancestors that were much more nutrient dense—but also smaller, more fibrous, less attractive, and less sweet.[8] The problem is that human beings prefer sweet, starchy, and tender foods that look nice and are pleasurable to eat. Agribusiness prefers larger fruits and vegetables that boost crop yields. Over ten thousand years of agricultural development, farmers and plant breeders have cultivated the biggest, sweetest, and mildest-tasting plants and removed any strong flavors. That's what sells!

However, this process has led to a dramatic loss of nutrients, fiber, antioxidants, and phytochemicals and a huge increase in sugar. Many of the most beneficial bionutrients have a sour, bitter, or astringent taste. These beneficial nutrients, which are protective against modern diseases such as heart disease and cancer, are what we need to try to recover and get more of through our modern-day fruits and vegetables.

Let's examine the phytonutrient difference between wild and contemporary plants, picking apples as an example. What do you think would be the percentage difference in phytochemicals between 1 ounce of wild apples and 1 ounce of modern apples? You know by now that the wild fruit has more nutrients, but what percent more? 20? 50? 100? 1,000? In fact, wild apples from Nepal were found to have *475 times* more nutrients ounce for ounce than one of our modern apples (a staggering difference of 47,500 percent)![9]

A striking 2009 study found that eating one Golden Delicious apple a day for a month led to increased levels of triglycerides and a subtype of LDL (low-density lipoprotein) cholesterol.[10] The adage "an apple a day keeps the doctor away" no longer holds true, especially with our modern-day apples. This is because the Golden Delicious apple, which happens to be the world's top-selling apple, is so high in sugar and low in phytonutrients that it may in fact be harmful to health.

Clearly the old advice to "eat more fruits and vegetables" is outdated. Also, you can't just go out and buy wild apples, unless you visit rural Nepal. You need to know which fruits and vegetables to purchase in today's world and how to maximize the nutritional "bang for your buck." In this chapter, I cover not just which plants to eat but how to store and prepare them in order to maximize nutrient density.

Let us begin by reviewing some general principles:

1. The more deeply and intensely colored a fruit or vegetable is, the more phytonutrients it contains. Darker colors such as red, purple, orange, black, and blue are usually a direct consequence of high phytochemical levels.
2. Most of a fruit or vegetable's antioxidants, which are part of its defense and repair mechanisms, are in the skin and just below the surface. Remember that antioxidants are how a plant protects itself against sun damage, traumatic injury, insects, and other causes; because the surface of a fruit is the most vulnerable to these external forces, it is near the skin and surface that the plant's antioxidants are concentrated. This is true for potatoes, carrots, oranges, avocados, and many other fruits and vegetables. Whenever possible, eat the peels, and especially the flesh that's right under the peel.
3. Sometimes frozen or canned produce can be as good as or better than fresh. The heat in the canning process can make nutrients more available—for example, this holds true with canned blueberries.
4. How you store, prepare, and cook food can dramatically affect its nutrient content. We'll go through specific examples below.
5. Vegetables lose nutrients with time once you bring them home. Therefore, eat the foods that lose their nutrients most rapidly first. Examples of such foods are artichokes, asparagus, broccoli, kale, leeks, lettuce, and spinach.

## Green Leafy Vegetables

Vegetables are alive. After harvest, they continue to consume oxygen and produce carbon dioxide. The scientific term for this is "respiratory rate." Some, like green leafy vegetables, have a high respiratory rate, and others, like potatoes, have a low respiratory rate. The point is that they are breathing. Start thinking about the vegetables you buy and bring home as living things—because in fact, they are, and this will remind you to pay more attention to how they are stored.

Ayurveda believes that all living things, including plants, have an essential substance known as prana, or life force. Whenever a living thing is born or created, it takes on prana. When it dies, prana leaves its form. This concept of life force is common to many Eastern traditions, where it is known by different names, such as *qi* in China and *ki* in Japan.

A living plant still in the soil is full of prana. As soon as the plant is harvested, the prana starts to slowly decline. Basically, as the plant is slowly dying, prana is leaving it. The steps you can take to maintain the freshness of fruits and vegetables, which are discussed below, also help to preserve their prana. This is one of the many reasons why homegrown fruits and vegetables are incredibly nutritious. There is very little loss of nutrients or prana before the food gets into your kitchen and onto your dinner plate. Compare this with the typical fruit or vegetable that travels hundreds or even thousands of miles from the farm before reaching the grocery store—the dissipation of nutrients is measurable, and the loss of prana is immense.

Green leafy vegetables, such as lettuce, because of their rapid respiratory rate, tend to lose nutrients quickly with the passage of time. If you store lettuce or greens in an airtight bag, after a few days the leaves will die from lack of oxygen, and their nutrients will break down and be gone. If you store lettuce without any covering, it is exposed to so much oxygen that it respires rapidly, using up all its antioxidants in the process. The best approach is somewhere in the middle, allowing the leaves access to some oxygen so they can breathe at the correct rate. Store leafy green vegetables in your refrigerator's crisper drawer in a plastic bag that has several evenly spaced holes poked in it. This allows in just enough oxygen but not so much that the vegetable respires too rapidly and loses its antioxidants.

Before storing leafy greens in your fridge, there is a quick, easy step that will immediately double the level of antioxidants in the vegetables: simply tear up the lettuce into smaller pieces. Referred to as "lettuce wounding" by researchers, this process doubles its antioxidant value.[11] The plant responds like it is being attacked by an insect and produces a burst of phytonutrients to fend off the intruder—you can benefit from this beneficial multiplication in antioxidants. It's like eating four servings of vegetables instead of two. This process hastens their decay, so you want to eat them within two days.

It is popular these days to buy prepackaged, prewashed, and precut greens. While it is preferable to buy the greens whole and cut them yourself, this option is acceptable as long as you cook them right away. Because cutting the greens has already sped up the rate of respiration and decay, you want to consume the precut greens as quickly as possible.

Let's review some differences in nutrient density among commonly consumed leafy greens. Iceberg lettuce, the most commonly consumed lettuce in the United States, is nutritionally poor except as a fiber source. Instead, choose **arugula, romaine, radicchio, or dark green or red loose-leaf lettuce**. The more deeply and darkly colored the greens, the more beneficial phytonutrients they contain.

**Romaine lettuce** is a great alternative and is full of vitamins and minerals in addition to phytochemicals. It is an excellent source of vitamin A (in the form of carotenoids), vitamin K, folate, and molybdenum. In addition, romaine lettuce is a good source of manganese, potassium, biotin, vitamin $B_1$, copper, iron, and vitamin C. It also contains vitamin $B_2$, omega-3 fatty acids, vitamin $B_6$, phosphorus, chromium, magnesium, calcium, and pantothenic acid.

**Spinach** is a nutrient-dense food. Rich in vitamins and minerals, it is also loaded with health-promoting phytonutrients such as carotenoids (beta-carotene, lutein, and zeaxanthin) and flavonoids to provide you with powerful antioxidant protection. Instead of boiling—where you lose water-soluble nutrients into the boiling water—steam or sauté the spinach.

With all greens, consuming them with good fats, especially **olive oil**, makes the nutrients more bioavailable. Soybean oil, the base of most commercial salad dressings, is only one-seventh as effective as olive oil for this purpose. To absorb more phytochemicals, enjoy your greens with an olive oil–based dressing, or make your own dressing with olive oil, balsamic vinegar, and spices.

## Cruciferous Vegetables

Cruciferous vegetables, one of the healthiest types of vegetables, include the following:

| | |
|---|---|
| Arugula | Horseradish |
| Bok choy | Kale |
| Broccoli | Radishes |
| Brussels sprouts | Rutabaga |
| Cabbage | Turnips |
| Cauliflower | Wasabi |
| Collard greens | Watercress |

Crucifers are rich in phytochemicals, which seem to reduce the potential of carcinogens through their ability to beneficially modulate liver detoxification enzymes—they inhibit certain enzymes that normally activate carcinogens while also inducing other enzymes that dismantle active carcinogens. Therefore, they are one of the most powerful foods to reduce the risk of cancer.

One example of their effect on liver enzymes is the ability of one of the phytonutrients found in cruciferous vegetables, indole-3-carbinol (I3C), to beneficially support the metabolism of estrogen. The liver metabolizes estrogen into either 16-alpha-hydroxyestrogen or 2-hydroxyestrogen, with the former predisposing to cancer development and the latter believed to oppose cancer development; the ratio of these two estrogen derivatives is used as a biomarker for the risk of developing hormone-dependent cancers such as those of the uterus and breast. I3C promotes the conversion of estrogen to 2-hydroxyestrogen and decreases the amount of 16-alpha-hydroxyestrogen. This selective conversion into 2-hydroxyestrogen is one way that crucifers decrease cancer risk. (It is possible to test for relative levels of these estrogen metabolites using functional medicine.)

**Broccoli** is rich in healthy antioxidants called sulphorophanes, which are cancer-fighting compounds. Raw broccoli has twenty-five times more sulphorophanes than cooked. If cooking broccoli, steam or sauté for only a few minutes. Avoid boiling or overcooking. Broccoli has a high respiratory rate, so cook right away or store in a microperforated bag.

**Brussels sprouts** kill more human cancer cells than other crucifers in lab test-tube studies. It has a high respiratory rate, so cook right away or store in a microperforated bag.

**Cabbage** is the world's most popular vegetable. Red cabbage has six times the antioxidants of green cabbage. Cabbage has a low respiratory rate and can be stored in the crisper drawer for weeks.

**Kale** is one of the few vegetables available that matches the nutritional value of wild greens. If you had to choose one vegetable to eat more of, I would probably recommend kale. It has the highest density of phytonutrients per gram of any vegetable. Raw kale is most nutritious, but lightly steamed or sautéed kale is a good alternative. It has a high respiratory rate, so cook right away or store in a microperforated bag.

**Cauliflower** is rich in glucosinolates, beneficial sulfur-containing compounds that are cancer-fighting. Green, orange, or purple cauliflower is even higher in antioxidants than white cauliflower. It has a medium respiratory rate and stays nutritious for a week in the fridge.

## Root Crops

### Potatoes

- In the form of french fries, potatoes are America's most popular vegetable.
- The skin contains half the antioxidants of the entire potato.
- Potatoes tend to raise blood sugar very rapidly. However, the glycemic index of potatoes can be lowered by chilling them for twenty-four hours after they have been cooked. This transforms the starch into "resistant starch," which is digested and absorbed slowly and benefits your microbiome (resistant starch is discussed more in Chapter 5).

### Sweet potatoes

- Sweet potatoes have a lower glycemic index and more antioxidants than white potatoes.
- The skin is more nutritious than the flesh, so eat them whole with the skin.
- Purple- or red-fleshed varieties have the most phytochemicals. Purple sweet potatoes are absolutely delicious and have complex, deep flavors that remind me of red wine. The purple-fleshed sweet potato's anthocyanins—primarily peonidins and cyanidins—have important antioxidant properties and anti-inflammatory properties.

- All root vegetables have a low respiratory rate and store well without loss of nutrients.

## Carrots

- A ten-year study from the Netherlands about carrot intake and risk of heart disease found that carrots were the most protective against heart disease among all the vegetables tested.[12]
- Carrots are better for you when cooked and eaten with oil. Heat breaks down tough cell walls and makes nutrients more bioavailable. Beta-carotene is a fat-soluble nutrient that needs to be eaten with fat for maximum absorption.
- Whole carrots have more nutrients than baby carrots. Once a carrot is cut, it begins to lose nutrients. Cooking a carrot whole and then cutting it into pieces preserves 30 percent more of its nutrients.
- Cooked uncut whole carrots with olive oil give you eight times more beta-carotene than a similar amount of raw baby carrots.
- Confirming the benefits of carrots for vision, researchers at the University of California at Los Angeles determined that women who consume carrots at least twice per week—in comparison to women who consume carrots less than once per week—have significantly lower rates of the eye disease glaucoma.

## Beets

- **Beet greens** have even more antioxidants than the roots and are the richest food source of betaine, a phytochemical that supports the liver, protects cells from environmental stress, and may reduce inflammation.
- **Beet juice** was found to enhance athletic performance and was consumed by a number of Olympic athletes recently. Red beets are more nutritious than yellow or white beets.
- An unheralded superfood, beets have fifty times more antioxidant activity than carrots. They are rich in cancer-fighting compounds called betalains, unique antioxidants that are not found in any other plants.

## Garlic

- Garlic is antibacterial, antiviral, and anticarcinogenic Allicin, the main sulfur-based active ingredient, is made in garlic when two substances in garlic that are stored in separate compartments are mixed together. However, it takes about ten minutes for this process to occur.
- To maximize nutritional benefits, **prepare garlic the following way**: Crush, mince, or mash the garlic and then wait for ten minutes. Then you may either consume the garlic raw or sauté or fry the garlic (without destroying the beneficial compounds) and still get all its health benefits. Do not cook it right after crushing.

## Onions

- The more pungent the onion, the better it is for you. Cooking onions increases their antioxidant value and makes the antioxidants more bioavailable than in raw onions.
- **Shallots** are highly nutritious vegetables that have six times more phytonutrients than the typical onion. They are smaller versions of onions that are closer to wild onions.
- **Green onions** (also known as scallions) are the closest to wild onions and have an astonishing 140 times more phytonutrients than common white onions. Incorporate these nutrient-dense wonders liberally in your diet.

## Tomatoes

- Wild tomatoes used to be much smaller. Smaller tomatoes are closer genetically to these wild ancestors and are therefore more nutritious.
- Diminutive cherry tomatoes have up to twelve times the lycopene of larger beefsteak tomatoes.
- Cooking tomatoes for thirty minutes can double their lycopene content by breaking down cell walls and transforming the lycopene into a form that is easier to absorb.
- Processed tomatoes are the richest sources of lycopene. Tomato paste has up to ten times more lycopene than raw tomatoes.

## Legumes

There is a lot of controversy about whether legumes were truly a part of ancestral diets (short answer: they probably were, based on anthropological research). However, they can be difficult to digest because of certain compounds that they contain, such as lectins and phytates. For people without digestive issues who can handle them, legumes are rich in antioxidants, fiber, and beneficial phytochemicals. Despite some issues with bioavailability because of lectins and phytates, legumes still offer a cornucopia of nutrients that can be absorbed. Therefore, if you tolerate them without any issue, legumes can be a beneficial addition to your diet. You may be surprised to see some of the following statistics about legumes:

- According to a USDA study, lentils have more antioxidants than blueberries.
- In a 2011 study of top antioxidant-rich foods in the United States, canned kidney beans ranked first. Canned pinto beans were second.
- Canned beans, especially black beans, lentils, kidney, and pinto beans, are very high in antioxidants; their nutrients are not destroyed during the canning process. Frozen legumes are less nutritious.
- Chickpeas and green peas are relatively low in antioxidant activity.
- If you are starting from scratch with dry legumes, be sure to soak them in water for twelve to twenty-four hours before cooking. Research has found that soaking at room temperature for eighteen hours or at 140°F for three hours eliminates between 30 to 70 percent of phytic acid, a substance that reduces our absorption of minerals such as calcium, iron, zinc, and magnesium and inhibits digestion.[13]
- If you simmer lentils in water, 70 percent of the antioxidants end up in the cooking liquid. Don't discard! Steaming or pressure-cooking lentils is a better alternative.

# Facts about Fruits

## Oranges

What part of an orange is the richest in antioxidants? The pith, which is the white covering just under the skin (again, the part below the peel is the most nutritious). Try to leave some of it on the orange when peeling it.

- **Navel oranges**, despite their sweet taste, are a low-glycemic nutrient-dense fruit.
- **Cara cara oranges** have a pinkish flesh and are rich in lycopene. They have three times as many antioxidants as conventional navel oranges.
- **Blood oranges** are also more nutritious than navel oranges and have blood red flesh that is rich in anthocyanins. These are very popular in Italy.
- Orange juice with pulp retained is higher in antioxidants than filtered juice.

## Apples

The low-nutrient Golden Delicious is the top-selling apple in the United States and worldwide! Choose a different apple that has more nutrients. Try to purchase organic, as apples are often high in pesticide residues.

- The skin of an apple is densely packed with nutrients, so always eat the skin. In animal studies, extracts from peeled apples inhibited the growth of human cancer cells by 14 percent, but extracts from unpeeled apples blocked the growth by 45 percent.
- **Granny Smith apples** have more nutrients than red apples. Braeburn, Gala, McIntosh, and Honeycrisp apples are rich in phytonutrients; among the least nutritious varieties are Golden Delicious, Ginger Gold, and Pink Lady.
- Deeply pigmented, more intensely colored apples tend to have the most phytochemicals. Therefore, try to choose the most colorful fruit within a given variety.
- Choose cloudy rather than clear apple juice and get four times as many phytonutrients.

## Peaches and nectarines

The skin has three times more phytonutrients per ounce than the flesh, so always eat the skins. Peaches and nectarines are exceptions to the shop-by-color rule, which states that the more colorful fruits and vegetables are, the more nutritious.

- **White-fleshed peaches** have up to six times the antioxidants as yellow-fleshed varieties.

- **Red-fleshed peaches** are the highest in antioxidants.
- Similarly, **white-fleshed nectarines** have several times the antioxidants as yellow-fleshed nectarines.

## Plums

Dark colored plums are rich in anthocyanins, an important class of antioxidants. **Red, purple, or black** plums are more nutritious than their lighter colored cousins. Dried plums, commonly called **prunes**, are rich in antioxidants. One study found that consuming prunes daily helped strengthen bones and prevent osteoporosis.

## Grapes

- **Red and black grapes** have four times the antioxidants of green grapes.
- **Welch's Concord grape juice** has more antioxidants than almost all other juices including acai. It may help slow age-related memory loss, lower blood pressure, prevent cholesterol oxidation, and thin the blood—thereby reducing the risk of heart attack or stroke.

## Berries

### Blueberries

- In animal studies, blueberries have been shown to reverse the aging of brains, to prevent tumor formation, and to slow the growth of existing tumors. They may also lower blood pressure and improve cholesterol profiles. Dried berries are much lower in antioxidants.
- Eat fresh berries or drink 100 percent berry juice. Frozen blueberries are equally nutritious. Cooking or canning blueberries increases their antioxidant levels because the heat changes the chemical structure of the berries.

**Blackberries** are phenomenally nutritious. While they are often overshadowed by blueberries, blackberries are in fact higher in antioxidants. Moreover, they have up to 10 g of fiber per cup and are low-glycemic.

**Cranberries** are rich in antioxidants. Most of the antioxidants are destroyed during the drying process that makes dried cranberries. However, because cranberries are so high in antioxidants, the dried fruit is still fairly nutritious. Also, 100 percent cranberry juice is an excellent source of phytochemicals.

**Strawberries** have very high levels of antioxidants and anti-inflammatory nutrients. This explains why research suggests that strawberries can help reduce the risk of cardiovascular disease, improve regulation of blood sugar, and help prevent certain cancers.

## Other Fruits

**Avocados**, which are in fact considered fruits rather than vegetables, are rich in antioxidants. In addition to their heart-healthy fatty acid profile, they may help lower LDL cholesterol and favorably impact the HDL/LDL ratio, based on a study published in 2015.[14] Also, researchers found that most of the antioxidants lie in the darker flesh just underneath the skin, so be sure to consume all the flesh left on the peels after you unpeel the avocado.

**Papayas** are rich in carotenoids, a powerful class of antioxidants. Red-fleshed fruit is more nutrient-rich than fruit with gold or yellow flesh.

**Mangos** have five times more vitamin C than oranges, five times more fiber than pineapples, and more phytonutrients than papayas.

**Watermelon** is rich in phytochemicals and antioxidants, especially lycopene. **Honeydew melon** and **cantaloupe** are relatively low in phytochemicals but higher in sugar.

As you can see, there are many nutrient-dense options in fruits and vegetables that can more effectively provide phytochemicals than the fruits and vegetables you may be currently eating. Simply making a few changes can help you dramatically increase nutrient density and ensure that you are getting all the right nutrients you need to keep your body in optimal shape.

# CHAPTER 5
# HEAL THE GUT—HEAL THE BODY

Ayurveda declares that the foundation of good health is a healthy digestive tract. Research in Western medicine is also establishing that optimizing digestive function is indispensable for overall well-being. My approach is always to "heal the gut first." I treat a lot of patients with autoimmune disease, and they're often surprised when I tell them that 80 percent of their immune systems is in their gut and that I'm going to begin their treatment with a gut healing program (even if they don't have any digestive symptoms).

## Say Hello to Your Gut Bacteria

One of the key components of optimal digestion is having a healthy microbiome. Most human beings have around 100 trillion bacteria and "only" 10 trillion human cells—therefore, you are only 10 percent human, and 90 percent bacterial. We know that the microbiome is complex and may contain over a thousand different species in the healthy individual. Anaerobic bacteria (which do not require oxygen for growth) may comprise more than 90 percent of the bacterial species.

Research has revealed that gut bacteria play a critical role in a number of processes, including carbohydrate digestion, energy storage, maintaining the health of intestinal cells, enhancing immune function, and protecting against pathogenic organisms. In addition, gut flora imbalance is implicated in various chronic illnesses, including obesity, insulin resistance, and cardiovascular disease.

Some of the most exciting new research is about the role of healthy gut flora in weight loss. Certain bacteria can affect metabolic functions by changing cell signaling and affecting the body's creation of fat. There appears to be a change in the gut microbiome in obese people that corresponds to changes in weight. More research is needed to understand these interconnections, but it is clear that the microbiome plays a fundamental role in metabolic balance and obesity.

## Microbiome Assessment Quiz

Take the following quiz to determine the relative health of your microbiome. Answer yes or no to the following statements:

- I was born via vaginal delivery and my mother was not on antibiotics during labor.
- I was breast-fed for at least one year by my mother.
- I received no more than two courses of antibiotics before the age of three.
- I have not taken antibiotics within the past one year.
- I do not use any antibacterial soaps or hand sanitizers.
- I grew up on a farm or in a rural area or in a developing country until the age of ten.
- I currently eat a variety of fermented foods on most days.
- I mostly drink water that is purified by reverse osmosis or other technology that can remove antibiotics from the water supply.
- I avoid feedlot-raised and factory-farmed meat, poultry, and fish.
- I am not under extreme stress and practice some type of mind-body stress reduction technique regularly.
- I eat a diet that's rich in both soluble and insoluble fiber as well as prebiotic foods (see page 84 for a list of prebiotic foods).
- I don't have any digestive symptoms such as heartburn, bloating, excessive gas, constipation, or diarrhea.

*How Did You Do?*
Count up the number of "Yes" answers that you have.

**Score: 12.** Congratulations! You likely have a vital and robust microbiome. Of course, there are other factors that could negatively affect the microbiome, but most likely you have a predominantly healthy balance of gut bacteria.

**Score: 9-11.** This is a good score. You have a lot of positive things in your favor to support the health of your microbiome. You want to continue working to maintain and possibly strengthen your gut bacteria.

**Score: 8 or below.** Your microbiome may have been adversely affected by the presence of negative factors such as antibiotic use or the absence of positive factors such as vaginal birth or breast-feeding. You can definitely improve your microbiome through the strategies outlined at the end of this chapter.

## The Destruction of the Human Microbiome

A number of factors have been shown to adversely affect the microbiome. These include reduced breast-feeding rates, low-fiber diets, increased consumption of processed foods, widespread use of antibiotics, emotional stress, and environmental toxins. Over the years, increased use of antibiotics in livestock, overprescribing of antibiotics by physicians, sterilization of our drinking water, reduced exposure to farm animals and microbe-rich environments, increased use of antibacterial soap and cleansers, and improved sanitation of the environment has led to dramatic decreases in the microbial diversity that we are exposed to while growing up.

## The Consequences of Antibiotic Overuse

While antibiotics were one of the most important advances in medicine in the twentieth century, it is clear now that antibiotics are being overused and overprescribed in both outpatient clinics and hospitals.[1] Dr. Martin Blaser describes in his book *Missing Microbes* how the overuse of antibiotics may have unintended adverse health consequences for humanity.[2] As a result of all of these factors, there is strong evidence that the human microbiome has declined significantly in biodiversity and quality over the past century.

In some ways, there has been a perfect storm of factors that could have the most detrimental effect possible on the microbiome. Some believe that this is an important factor in the rise of allergies and autoimmune disease such as celiac disease, rheumatoid arthritis, asthma, and Hashimoto's thyroid disease—the incidence of autoimmune disease is strongly correlated with higher levels of development and socioeconomic status (where antibiotic use is generally higher).

## Antibiotics in Meat—Imperceptible but Toxic

One of the biggest areas where antibiotics are overused is in modern factory farms, which use up to 70 to 80 percent of all antibiotics sold in the United States; not only are antibiotics used to prevent infections in the crowded, unsanitary conditions in modern feedlots and CAFOs (Confined Animal Feeding Operations), they are also given to animals to help them gain weight more quickly.[3] Therefore, the bulk of our commercial meat, milk, and egg supply is tainted with antibiotics; in fact, these foods are allowed a certain upper limit of antibiotic content, although legal limits are exceeded 9 percent of the time.[4]

This is why studies have shown that vegetarian diets seem to be more beneficial in some ways for our microbiome—conventional meat products may promote the growth of pathogenic bacteria through antibiotics that harm our beneficial bacteria as well as resistant organisms that are present in the meat as a result of antibiotic overuse in animals.[5]

In addition, there is a possible link between colon cancer and gut bacteria. Studies have connected a group of enzymes, including beta-glucuronidase, to colon cancer; people who eat conventional meat appear to have higher levels of these enzymes than people who are vegetarian.[6] These cancer-related enzymes seem to originate from pathogenic bacteria in the intestines, primarily as toxins produced by these bacteria.

This may explain the possible association between colon cancer and red meat based on various studies.[7] The problem is not really the meat itself but the negative effect of antibiotic-laced conventional red meat on gut bacteria and the presence of pathogenic bacteria in meat resulting from antibiotic overuse—both of which can cause an increase in cancer-related enzymes.

Interestingly, the levels of these enzymes seem to fall significantly following supplementation with certain probiotics, suggesting that the beneficial bacteria in probiotics can reduce the levels of pathogenic bacteria that are producing these enzymes.[8] The unavoidable conclusion is that factory-farmed animal protein is likely to be harmful to your microbiome, and that's why I recommend avoiding it. If you are going to eat meat, I recommend eating pasture-raised organic meat and eschewing farmed fish in favor of wild-caught fish.

## What If I Have To Take Antibiotics?

I am not categorically opposed to antibiotics. There may be times when they are medically indicated and even lifesaving. What can you do to protect your microbiome if you have to take antibiotics? The first thing is to definitely take a good broad-spectrum probiotic *as soon as you begin to take* the antibiotic. Taking probiotics simultaneously with antibiotics helps to minimize the damage to your beneficial bacteria and may reduce side effects such as antibiotic-associated diarrhea. Taking probiotics after you complete your course of antibiotics is useful but does not address the disruption of your gut bacteria during the course of antibiotics. Minimizing the duration of time that a person's microbiome is disrupted is critical, and the best way to do this is to begin the probiotics at the same time as starting antibiotics. It is helpful to space apart the probiotic dosage from the antibiotics by at least two hours. For, example if you are on a twice-daily antibiotic, you could take it with breakfast and dinner, and take your probiotic supplement with lunch and at bedtime. In terms of the specific probiotic supplement, a broad-spectrum blend that contains the beneficial yeast *Saccharomyces boulardii* would be especially helpful. Since *Saccharomyces boulardii* is a yeast and not a bacteria, it is immune to the effects of antibiotics and can be helpful in stabilizing your gut flora.

The second strategy is to ensure that you are consuming fermented foods such as sauerkraut, kefir, kimchi, and/or yogurt once or twice a day while you are on the antibiotics. Fermented foods are rich sources of beneficial bacteria and fungi.

Lastly, consuming more prebiotic foods, which feed the growth of your beneficial bacteria, can be helpful. Prebiotic foods can be complemented by prebiotic supplements that also specifically nourish your microbiome. (Prebiotics are discussed later in this chapter.)

## The Hygiene or "Old Friends" Hypothesis

What are some of the consequences of this radical change in the human microbiome? The hygiene hypothesis states that as public sanitation, toilets, clean drinking water, and other "hygiene" measures became more prevalent, the incidence of diseases involving abnormalities of the immune system such as autoimmune disease began to increase. This is an oversimplification, and one of the original proponents of the hygiene hypothesis, Graham Rook, has renamed it the "old friends" hypothesis.

This idea states that these so-called "old friends" are a specific group of organisms, such as parasites, key bacteria in our microbiome, and non-parasitic mycobacteria (called saprophytes) that have co-evolved with human beings over the past eons; before widespread sanitation and pervasive antibiotic use, these organisms were present in our food, water, and within our bodies throughout our entire lives.[9] Because we were constantly exposed to them, we evolved to "live with them."

Did our immune systems in fact evolve expecting these "old friends" to dampen them? That's the essence of the "old friends" hypothesis. If our immune systems were hypersensitive and always reacting to these organisms that were inevitably present within us and around us, the body would be in a constant state of inflammation, which would be very harmful and maladaptive. Moreover, it is often a survival strategy of "old friends" to depress and put a brake on the immune system in order to ensure their own continuance and survival; by necessity they had to suppress our immune systems so that they could live in our bodies for long periods without being killed. If they were unable to quiet and down-regulate the immune system, the human host would eradicate them and prevent them from establishing a long-term home in the human body.

## Leaning into the Wind

The way this process occurred is explained by Rook as follows—"evolution turns the inevitable into a necessity"—which means that if something cannot be avoided, it will be incorporated into daily function and physiology and eventually become something that the body expects to find in the environment and not have to provide intrinsically.[10] Basically, one could use the metaphor of a person who is leaning into the wind. In this case, the wind is the vast number of "old friends" that human immune systems have been exposed to over the previous tens of thousands of years. Since the microbial "wind" has always been blowing for most of human evolution, human immune systems have evolved in response to lean slightly forward, effectively being just a bit overactive. The person who is leaning slightly forward but held in balance by the power of the wind is like the immune system that tends to be hyperactive but is restrained by the parasites and other microbes; when the wind is taken away, the person falls down—that is, the immune system gets out of balance and is no longer held in check, potentially contributing to the rise of autoimmune diseases.[11]

In the same manner, our resident "ancient organisms" such as *H. pylori* have evolved over eons to suppress our immune system's inflammatory response so that they can ensure their own survival. Specifically, *H. pylori,* when present in the stomach, attracts to the local tissues a large number of T-regulatory cells, which modify and suppress inflammation; T-regulatory cells (which can be thought of as the police officers of the immune system) are important for keeping a brake on the immune system and reducing overzealous inflammation, and may through their suppressive functions protect the immune system from reacting to other substances as commonly occurs in asthma, allergies, and other autoimmune conditions.[12]

Notably, chronic stress has also been shown to have a harmful effect on the gut bacteria, in addition to various other negative effects on the digestive system. When all these factors contribute to negatively affect the microbiome, they can lead to a condition known as leaky gut syndrome, one of the most common imbalances that I see in my patients.

## The Start of Illness—Leaky Gut Syndrome

What is leaky gut syndrome? Normally, intestinal cells are bunched together so that nothing slips by them. They have connections with each other that link tightly, just like the fingers on your hands when you interlace them together. In leaky gut syndrome, these connections between intestinal cells expand and create little gaps. This leads to increased intestinal permeability, which is the definition of leaky gut syndrome.

When the gut exhibits increased permeability, partially digested food particles can slip between the intestinal cells into the blood. This can be exacerbated if you have low digestive enzymes (something I see commonly in my patients) and are already not breaking down your food properly. The immune system does not recognize these strange-looking, partially digested proteins and creates antibodies to attack them. This is the first step in the development of food sensitivities, as the immune system begins to react to foods that it did not react to previously.

What causes leaky gut syndrome? Changes in the gut microbiome are definitely one of the key contributing factors. These include overgrowth of harmful bacteria (called bacterial dysbiosis), declines in healthy gut bacteria, or other infections such as viruses, fungi, or parasites. Also, inflammatory bowel disease such as ulcerative colitis or Crohn's disease leads to colonic inflammation and leaky gut. Lastly, certain food sensitivities (such as gluten sensitivity) can predispose one to the development of leaky gut syndrome, which then leads to worsening food sensitivities through a vicious circle.

Why is leaky gut a problem? The reason is that as food sensitivities worsen, the immune system sends out inflammatory chemicals and killer cells to attack the perceived enemies. Certain chemicals known as cytokines are produced in greater quantity, and these can have damaging effects on surrounding tissues. These same cytokines can subsequently attack other organs such as, for example, those of the nervous system, causing various mental or neurological symptoms. The hyperactive immune system can then mistakenly attack the body's own tissues, predisposing one to autoimmune disease. In fact, some scientists believe that it's not possible to have an autoimmune disease without some degree of leaky gut syndrome.

## How to Heal Leaky Gut Syndrome

How can you improve intestinal permeability and resolve leaky gut? The first step is identifying and removing any triggers that may be contributing to leaky gut syndrome. The Paleovedic Detox helps you eliminate the most common offending foods. If you have any gastrointestinal symptoms, it may be beneficial to consult a functional medicine practitioner to have some testing done to evaluate your microbiome, measure digestive enzymes, screen for infections, and treat any imbalances that may be contributing.

Ensuring that you have good levels of digestive enzymes is a good way to start. An Ayurvedic tip is to chew a small piece of ginger dipped in lemon juice before meals. Another approach is to consume a small quantity of bitters (alcohol infused with bitter herbs), such as Swedish bitters or Angostura bitters, before eating. Finally, a teaspoon of apple cider vinegar in eight ounces of water before meals can also stimulate your enzymes.

There are a few ways to restore the normal permeability of the intestinal barrier. An inexpensive age-old remedy, bone broth, is actually helpful for this purpose. Its gelatin content and minerals are helpful in repairing leaky gut.

L-glutamine, an amino acid found naturally in the body, can often help with treating leaky gut. In supplement form, take at least 4 g per day in two divided doses. If you're not eating fish regularly, 1,000 mg per day of combined EPA and DHA in supplement form can provide beneficial nutrition for intestinal cells. There are a number of other herbs and supplements that can be beneficial in leaky gut—please consult your local functional medicine practitioner.

## Probiotics vs. Prebiotics

Altering the microbiome in a beneficial way can support gut function. In principle, there are two major strategies for influencing the flora. One is the use of living bacteria taken orally, which must survive the gastrointestinal tract to be active in the colon. This can be through either foods that contain good bacteria or probiotic supplements. The second strategy is through food, specifically using dietary ingredients known as prebiotics that are indigestible, reach the colon, and can be used by health-promoting colonic bacteria.

Studies show that prebiotics are the more effective way to quantitatively increase the number of beneficial bacteria in your microbiome. Probiotics have a wide variety of benefits but function more as immunomodulators and a support to your own beneficial bacteria rather than long-term quantitative boosters of your own microbiome; supplemental probiotics typically stay in your gut only during the period of supplementation but then are gradually excreted and typically no longer detectable after about two weeks.[13] Therefore, supplemented probiotics rarely become permanent residents of the microbiome; this does not detract in any way from their potential beneficial effects, however.

The microbiome of a child typically reaches a stable, permanent state that resembles the adult microbiome by around the age of three.[14] Resident strains of probiotics are likely those that have been present over many generations within our families, and the same strains that we received from our mothers are likely the ones that we will pass on to our children, thus making it likely that we have probiotic strains that are unique to us and, to some degree, shared among our family members.

## Your Appendix Is Not Useless

Interestingly, some research suggests that the appendix—formerly thought to be a vestigial organ with no real purpose currently in the human body—may play an important role in our microbiome. There is evidence that the appendix incubates or stores a "library" of resident bacterial species and has the capacity to reintroduce and reinoculate the intestines with specific strains of bacteria when needed.[15] Further research is needed to investigate this theory, but it may explain the connection of the appendix with lymphatic tissue, which constitutes part of the immune system.

## Fermented Foods

Fermented foods such as sauerkraut, kimchi, and kefir are rich sources of beneficial bacteria and if prepared correctly may even contain more probiotics than probiotic supplements. Other fermented foods include yogurt, crème fraiche, miso, *natto*, and *kombucha*. Many traditional cultures used fermentation or pickling to preserve foods before the advent of refrigeration and consumed various fermented foods.

South Indian cuisine includes *dosa* and *idli*, which are made from a fermented mixture of rice and lentils, and *appam*, which is made from fermented rice and coconut milk. *Lassi* is a widely available fermented dairy beverage that is typically consumed after meals. India features a rich variety of traditional fermented foods that are derived from many different food sources, including *khalpi* (cucumber), *dhokla* (rice and lentil), *sinki* (radish), *ghungruk* (green leafy vegetables), *kanjika* (millet), and *iromba* (fish).[16] African cuisine also features a variety of fermented foods, such as bread made from fermenting grains like sorghum or teff.

Fermented foods include:

- Sauerkraut
- Kimchi
- Kvass
- Pickled ginger
- Pickled cucumbers
- Yogurt (if you tolerate dairy)
- Lassi
- Coconut yogurt
- Crème fraiche
- Miso
- Natto
- Kombucha
- Kefir (a fermented beverage made from either dairy or nondairy sources)

## The Gut-Brain Axis

The regular consumption of a variety of fermented foods helps maintain a robust and diverse microbiome. In addition to digestive benefits, fermented foods can support cognitive function because there is a strong gut-brain connection. A randomized, double-blind, placebo-controlled trial showed that supplemental probiotics have the ability to positively impact mood and mental health status after just six weeks of intervention.[17] Another study found that increased intake of fermented foods is linked with reduced social anxiety.[18] Studies like these demonstrate the power of the gut-brain axis and the importance of digestive health for mental health. This connection may be mediated by serotonin, a neurotransmitter critical for mood and sleep that is produced in larger quantities in the gut than in the brain. There are over twenty major neurotransmitters made in the intestines, which are influenced by the microbiome and may affect our mental and emotional state. The vagus nerve, which carries signals bidirectionally from the gut to the brain, also plays an important role in this connection. In fact, the gut is widely known as "the second brain," rivaling our primary brain in complexity and sophistication. I have seen depression or anxiety improve in some of my patients just after doing a gut-healing protocol.

## Case—Sphincter of Oddi Dysfunction

Rebecca was a fifty-two-year-old management consultant who had developed unexplained abdominal pain a few years earlier. She was eventually seen at

Stanford and after numerous tests was diagnosed with a rare condition known as sphincter of Oddi dysfunction. The sphincter of Oddi controls the release of enzymes from the pancreas and liver into the intestine to help with digestion. For unclear reasons, it sometimes malfunctions, causing severe abdominal pain and food intolerance. Rebecca did not improve despite taking multiple prescribed drugs for over a year and was only able to eat five or six different foods. She was recommended to undergo surgical treatment, which carries a high risk of complications. She came to see me hoping to avoid surgery.

After evaluating Rebecca, I put her on a "Gut Repair Program" with anti-inflammatory herbs, gut-healing supplements, fermented foods, and foods rich in prebiotics. After three months, her pain had subsided, and she gradually reintroduced different foods—she said she knew she was well when she had a four-course Thai dinner late one night and had no symptoms. She was surprised that a very specific dysfunction relating to the sphincter of Oddi could be addressed with such a program. I explained to her that the gut has a remarkable self-healing potential, and the right foods and supplements can help correct most imbalances.

## Prebiotic-rich Foods

Certain foods are rich in prebiotics, compounds that feed beneficial bacteria. These are mostly short chains of complex carbohydrates called oligosaccharides. The most common types of oligosaccharides are inulin, fructo-oligosaccharides (FOS), galactooligosaccharides (GOS), and transgalactooligosaccharides (TOS); inulin and FOS are primarily found in vegetables, especially root vegetables, while GOS and TOS are derived from dairy products.[19] Interestingly, these prebiotics are also inhibitory to potentially pathogenic bacterial species such as salmonella, shigella, campylobacter, and listeria, which tend to thrive on refined sugars as opposed to complex oligosaccharides. They also appear to be beneficial for increasing the absorption of certain nutrients, such as calcium.[20]

GOS is present in breast milk in high concentrations and is supportive of the infant's microbiome. Colonic bacteria ferment GOS, producing short-chain fatty acids such as n-butyrate, one of the main energy sources for intestinal cells. Two groups of beneficial bacteria—the bifidobacteria and lactobacilli—seem to thrive on GOS. Apart from prebiotic effects, GOS appears also to reduce the ability of pathogens to breach the intestinal wall and have direct interaction with immune cells, thereby helping defend against infection.[21]

Prebiotic-rich foods include:

- Garlic
- Onions
- Bananas
- Oats
- Jerusalem artichoke
- Asparagus
- Leeks
- Chicory
- Beets
- Sweet potatoes
- Yams
- Yucca
- Cassava
- Taro
- Lotus root

Other sources of prebiotics that you can incorporate in moderation if you tolerate them include dairy products, legumes such as black beans and lentils, and other whole grains. Note that you may be better off avoiding certain foods, such as whole grains or legumes, for other reasons, as discussed earlier. Sometimes you may experience increased gas as a side effect of consuming increased quantities of prebiotic-rich foods. This is because the bacteria that are fermenting them in the colon may produce gas as a metabolic by-product.

Some foods, such as Jerusalem artichoke, which are very high in inulin, are notorious for causing increased abdominal gas. If this becomes problematic, simply reduce the quantity of the food that you are consuming. Over time, as your microbiome shifts and becomes increasingly efficient at metabolizing prebiotics, side effects such as gas should subside.

CAUTION: If you are suffering from an overgrowth of harmful bacteria (such as small intestinal bacterial overgrowth or bacterial dysbiosis), prebiotic-rich foods or supplements like resistant starch can make your symptoms worse. Consult with your functional medicine practitioner if you suspect that you have such a condition or if you have intolerable side effects from prebiotics.

## Resistant Starch

A special kind of insoluble fiber known as resistant starch can be especially effective as a prebiotic. Resistant starch refers to a type of starch that "resists" digestion by our enzymes but can be broken down and metabolized by bacteria. This increases the number of your beneficial bacteria and produces short-chain fatty acids, which are nourishing for intestinal cells.

Resistant starch also improves blood sugar parameters, increases insulin sensitivity, and may have other metabolic effects as well. There are a few sources of resistant starch.

Cooked and chilled potatoes are an excellent source. Any traditional potato, like white, brown, red, or even purple can be used for this purpose. Potatoes that have been cooked and then chilled in the refrigerator for twenty-four hours undergo a transformation that leads to the production of resistant starch. After twenty-four hours, the potatoes can be reheated without any loss or damage to the resistant starch. Potato salad could work well for this purpose.

Cooking and cooling white rice produces a modest amount of resistant starch. Scientists from Sri Lanka have found that if you add 2 teaspoons of coconut oil for each 1 cup of white rice while cooking, and then chill the cooked rice for twelve hours, you can significantly increase the resistant starch content and decrease the calories of the rice by at least 10 percent.[22] Parboiled white rice has more resistant starch and fiber than regular white rice. Green, unripe plantains and green bananas also have appreciable amounts of resistant starch.

## Using Resistant Starch Supplements

Potato starch (not potato flour) is an excellent source of resistant starch. This is widely available in most grocery stores and online. Common brands include Bob's Red Mill or Anthony's Potatoes (Organic). It is a fine white powder that is tasteless and dissolves easily in water. If you are using it as a resistant starch supplement, the trick is to consume it raw. If you cook potato starch, it will be absorbed and metabolized in your body; when you eat it raw, you won't be able to derive any nutrition from it (therefore, it is not a significant source of calories), but your gut bacteria will.

If you are going to take it as a supplement, I would recommend starting very slowly, perhaps with a quarter teaspoon dissolved in four ounces of water once per day after a meal. Sometimes people may have digestive symptoms such as gas or bloating as their gut bacteria are changing. If this occurs, try lowering the dose. If you are someone who is sensitive to supplements, I recommend starting with a lower dose, like an eighth of a teaspoon, and working up in increments of an eighth of a teaspoon. If you still don't tolerate it, consult with a functional medicine practitioner. If you tolerate a quarter teaspoon, stay on this dose for three days, and monitor for any side effects, like gas, bloating, or change in stool consistency. If no major side effects occur, gradually increase by a quarter teaspoon every three days up to a dosage of one tablespoon per day. I would consume it for a maximum of one month and then check with your practitioner for further recommendations.

Green plantain, which can be purchased as a food or a supplement, can be beneficial as another source of resistant starch. Again, the trick is to consume it raw. One option is to dehydrate plantains to make chips and consume them that way. An alternative is to purchase green plantain flour. Again, if you are going to take it as a supplement, I would recommend starting very slowly, perhaps with a quarter teaspoon (or an eighth of a teaspoon if you are sensitive) dissolved in four ounces of water once per day. Stay on this dose for three days to observe for any side effects, like gas, bloating, or change in stool consistency. If well tolerated, gradually increase by a quarter teaspoon every three days up to a dosage of one tablespoon per day. Other sources of resistant starch are green banana flour and cassava starch. Resistant starch supplements like potato starch can also be blended in with a smoothie or protein drink—any food product in which they are not heated will work.

## Case—Irritable Bowel Syndrome

Marcy was a thirty-seven-year-old mother of two who had struggled with irritable bowel syndrome for more than ten years. Despite having eliminated gluten and dairy products, she still struggled with daily bloating, abdominal pain, and diarrhea. She had seen multiple gastroenterologists who had performed almost every known GI test on her—all of which came back normal. I took a functional medicine approach with her, and testing identified low digestive enzymes, deficiency of beneficial bacteria, and yeast overgrowth. After a two-month "Gut Repair Program" with digestive enzymes, antifungal herbs, probiotics, and foods including bone broth and fermented foods, she reported about 80 percent improvement of her symptoms. Follow-up testing revealed persistent deficiency in certain beneficial bacterial strains that was targeted with prebiotics. After two more months, she surprised her gastroenterologists by reporting that she was symptom-free, a state she has maintained to this day. She was able to gradually wean off her supplements and use specific foods to keep her gut in good shape.

## Eat Sh*t and Live

There is one other, more extreme way to alter gut flora: fecal microbiota transplantation. This is where stool from a healthy donor is introduced into the digestive tract of the patient, typically either through a tube passed through the nose into the stomach or directly into the colon through enema or colonoscopy.[23] Because fecal transplant has been scientifically proven to be the best therapy for recurrent *Clostridium difficile* infection, even superior to the conventional treatment of multiple courses of powerful antibiotics, it has been approved by the FDA for this condition. *Clostridium difficile* (*C. diff*) is a harmful bacterium that can cause a serious gastrointestinal infection that leads to severe diarrhea and colitis. While this can be treated with antibiotics, the recurrence rate is high, and resistance to antibiotics develops quickly, often leading to treatment failure and potential complications including death; the presence of *C. diff* in hospitalized patients has a mortality rate close to 25 percent at one month.[24]

Remarkably, fecal microbiota transplantation consistently cures even the most refractory *Clostridium difficile* infections with success rates above 90 percent. This is far superior to any antibiotic. How does it work? It is thought that the beneficial bacteria in the donor stool inhibits *C. diff* directly and have immune system regulating responses that help eradicate the infection. While this is still considered an investigational treatment by the FDA, research is ongoing to see whether fecal transplants can be helpful in other conditions.

## How to Strengthen Your Microbiome

We used to say that "you are what you eat." Ayurveda would respond that "you are what you eat, digest, and absorb." By ensuring that you have a healthy digestive tract, including normal intestinal permeability and a robust microbiome, you can be certain that you are digesting and absorbing as many nutrients as possible from your diet. This will go a long way toward ensuring that a healthy diet will actually translate into optimal well-being.

Here are some steps you can take to build up a healthy microbiome:

- Eat at least two servings of various fermented foods on most days.
- Consume a diet that's rich in both soluble and insoluble fiber as well as resistant starch.
- Incorporate a variety of prebiotic-rich foods into your diet daily.
- Avoid unnecessary antibiotic use. Of course, appropriate antibiotics for genuine bacterial infections can be beneficial and even lifesaving.
- Avoid using antibacterial soaps or hand sanitizers.
- Practice a daily mind-body stress-reduction technique.
- Drink water that is purified by reverse osmosis or other technology that can remove antibiotics from water.
- Avoid feedlot-raised and factory-farmed meat, poultry, and fish. Eat only pasture-raised meat or wild-caught fish.
- If you tolerate dairy, consume certified organic dairy products, and avoid conventional dairy, which typically has antibiotic residues.
- Get a dog or cat. Seriously, any exposure to animals can be helpful in expanding the diversity of your microbiome.

# CHAPTER 6

# YOUR AYURVEDIC BODY TYPE—THE KEY TO CUSTOMIZATION

This chapter introduces Ayurveda, which offers an explanation of why different people require different diets, even if they are part of a population with very similar genetic makeup. It also provides detailed insights into how to individualize a dietary program for each person. Each of us has a different Ayurvedic body type, and a simple questionnaire will help you determine your body type and understand the optimal foods for each type.

## The Science of Life

First, let me tell you more about Ayurveda, which is named from the Sanskrit words "Ayu" meaning "life" and "Veda" meaning "science"—that is, "The Science of Life." Ayurveda is a holistic system of medicine that has a comprehensive approach to understanding the body. It can be traced back at least three thousand years, and is probably the oldest system of medicine in the world.

The Ayurvedic approach to science is different, although no less rigorous, than the allopathic paradigm. When I began studying Ayurveda in the late 1990s, I found Ayurvedic theory logical enough to satisfy my Western training.

## Understanding the Doshas

The foundation of Ayurveda is the concept of *doshas*, or physiological principles. You can think of the doshas as forces within the body that are responsible for all the physiological and psychological processes in your body and mind. There are three main doshas—vata (which you can think of as wind), pitta (equivalent to fire), and kapha (earth). The doshas are shifting constantly, due to diet, lifestyle, and environment. As long as they are balanced and working harmoniously together, good health is possible. When the doshas are imbalanced, disease results. Let us look at each of the doshas in more detail:

## Vata

- Vata is the subtle energy that governs all movement in the body, including respiration, heartbeat, nerve impulses, blood flow, and so forth.
- Like "wind," vata's qualities are light, cold, dry, and mobile.
- Associated with creativity and rapid thinking, but also fear, anxiety, and restlessness.

## Pitta

- The bodily heat-energy of metabolism, manifesting in digestion, absorption, temperature regulation.
- Like "fire," pitta is hot, sharp, penetrating, and intense.
- Linked with Agni, digestive capacity.
- Associated with intelligence and insight, but also anger, irritability, and frustration.

## Kapha

- The force that forms body structure and provides biological "strength," associated with bones, joints and ligaments, skin moisture, and joint lubrication.
- Like "mud," it is heavy, cool, slow, and damp.
- Associated with love and calmness, but also attachment, depression, and inertia.

# The 7 Dhatus or Tissues

In addition to the three doshas, there are seven *dhatus* or tissues that constitute the structure of the body. These include *rasa* (plasma and lymph), *rakta* (blood), *mamsa* (muscle), *medas* (fat), *asthi* (bone), *majja* (bone marrow and nerve tissue), and *shukra* (reproductive tissue). These tissues are also in a state of constant transformation and interplay, just like the doshas, and optimal dhatu status is essential for good health.

Because of three doshas and seven dhatus, a period of twenty-one days is considered to be especially significant and adequate for fundamental shifts to occur throughout the body. That is why the Paleovedic Detox, discussed in Chapter 12, is designed to be three weeks long.

## Every Person Is Unique

Every person is born with a distinct combination of doshas that comprises their constitution, which is as unique as a fingerprint. Nobody has exactly the same ratio of vata, pitta, and kapha. Also, each person manifests the qualities of their doshas in a slightly different way as a result of their personality and other factors. The goal in Ayurveda is to maintain your unique balance of doshas, which was determined at conception.

For example, let's say that you are 50 percent vata, 30 percent pitta, and 20 percent kapha (every person has at least a little bit of all three of doshas). Consequently, the optimal dosha balance that you want to strive for is 50 percent vata, 30 percent pitta, and 20 percent kapha, which is identical to your constitution. You are not trying to get equal amounts of all three doshas, which is a common misconception.

Using the same example, your primary dosha would be vata and your secondary dosha is pitta. As a rule of thumb, the primary dosha has the greatest tendency to increase and become imbalanced. Therefore, a vata person is more likely to experience a vata excess and thereby suffer vata-related disease. That is why the diet for each dosha has qualities and characteristics opposite to the dosha. For example, the qualities of the vata dosha are light, cold, and dry; the foods that are recommended as part of the vata diet are heavy, warm, and moist—both in terms of physical characteristics and subtle qualities.

In general, "like attracts like," and this may or may not be beneficial depending on the dosha. For example, pitta body types tend to love hot, spicy food, although that is potentially aggravating for their pitta dosha in excess. They might do better with spices that are considered cooling, such as cumin, coriander, fennel, and cilantro. The typical recommended diet for pitta people contains foods that would be considered to have cooling properties.

Interestingly, this appears to extend beyond dietary preferences. In my practice, I see many kapha patients who love to relax and enjoy sitting quietly, whereas intense, vigorous, and stimulating activities would be beneficial for them. Many of my vata patients take on too much activity and tend to crave fast action and new experiences, and I remind them to slow down and incorporate more downtime and relaxation. Pittas are attracted to competitive sports that reward intensity and aggression, whereas more restorative exercise would be balancing for them. Of course, these are generalizations, but I find it striking how often they are relevant to patients in my practice.

Ayurveda is able to take the science of prevention to the next level, by telling you what types of imbalances and diseases you are most prone to as a result of your specific body type. This enables you to anticipate potential illness and take corrective steps before it manifests. This is one reason I find Ayurveda to be so powerful.

## Eat Right for Your Body Type

Ayurveda recommends a different diet for each constitution, and so you would follow the diet recommended for your body type. Ayurveda also believes that the diet should be individualized based on season, environment, activity level, and overall goals. For example, each season is associated with a certain dosha; winter is a time when the excess cold can provoke vata, and the heat of summer can increase pitta. To learn about your body type and its recommended diet, please complete the following questionnaire.

## Ayurvedic Body Type Questionnaire

Each person is born with an Ayurvedic body type or prakriti. On each line, please choose the one answer that best describes you around age fifteen to twenty. Then, circle the answer in the appropriate column. At the bottom, please add up the totals from each column. The column with the highest score is your primary dosha, and the column with the second highest score is your secondary dosha.

## DETERMINE YOUR AYURVEDIC BODY TYPE

Ask a friend to help you if you like. For each row, select the column containing the words that best describe your true nature and qualities. All the words may not apply; you just want the closest fit. If two columns describe you equally well, circle both. Each answer corresponds to one point. At the bottom, please add up the totals from each column. The column with the highest score is your primary dosha, and the column with the second highest score is your secondary dosha.

| CHARACTERISTICS | VATA | PITTA | KAPHA |
|---|---|---|---|
| Body frame, bone structure | Slight, thin, delicate, bony with prominent joints | Moderate, medium sized; joints not particularly prominent | Broad, strong, heavy; bones and joints not prominent |
| Body weight | Underweight, lean, difficult to gain or weight often fluctuates | Moderate weight, strong metabolism, maintains steady weight | Overweight, very difficult to lose weight |
| Skin | Dry, rough, uneven or combination skin, chapped, cold | Fair or light skin, soft, oily; sensitive, burns easily; ruddy complexion; freckles or moles | Thick, soft, smooth, moist, cool |
| Hands | Long, thin fingers; rectangular palm | Medium-sized, slender fingers; square palm | Short, fleshy fingers; thick palm |
| Hair | Dry, rough, tends to break, curly, frizzy | Blonde, yellow or red; early gray or thinning or bald | Thick, full, dense, wavy, lustrous, oily |
| Tongue | Dry, thin, pale, cracked, tends to be tremulous | Pointed, tapering shape; intensely red color | Large for the mouth, thick, round tip, glossy |
| Eyes | Small; brown or black colored; flitting gaze, tends to blink a lot | Medium sized, light or pale colored; sharp, penetrating gaze | Large, round; blue or brown; steady gaze, does not blink much |

| CHARACTERISTICS | VATA | PITTA | KAPHA |
|---|---|---|---|
| Neck | Long, skinny; prominent Adam's apple | Medium in size, veins easily visible; less prominent Adam's apple | Short, broad, stout; Adam's apple not visible |
| Body temperature/ sweating | Often feels cold, especially hands and feet, doesn't sweat much | Usually warm, sweats easily and profusely | Not particularly hot or cold, may not sweat much |
| Temperature preference | Loves hot weather, doesn't mind humidity | Easily overheated, prefers cool climates, hates hot weather | Not disturbed by heat or cold, but prefers warm weather |
| Appetite | Variable, irregular, "eyes bigger than stomach"; cannot skip meals as becomes ravenous, must eat frequently | Very good appetite but can skip meals if needed; becomes irritable or gets heartburn when overly hungry | Fair appetite but doesn't have to eat regularly; can skip meals easily |
| Digestion and elimination | Variable, irregular digestion; tendency to constipation | Regular to fast digestion; tendency toward soft or loose stools, more than one bowel movement per day | Slow but steady digestion, regular consistent bowel movements |
| Physical activity/energy | Very active, but gets tired easily, extreme ups and downs, restless | Moderate, even, focused, has good stamina, enjoys pushing oneself and loves competition. | Lethargic, hard to get going, but has good endurance |
| Sleep | Light sleeper, moves a lot, restless, variable; needs a lot of sleep and feels tired if sleep-deprived | Moderate to sound sleeper, needs less sleep and can function with limited sleep if needed | Heavy sleeper, easily falls asleep; hard to wake up; does not need many hours |

| CHARACTERISTICS | VATA | PITTA | KAPHA |
|---|---|---|---|
| Mental disposition | Restless, active, creative. Learns quickly but also tends to forget quickly | Sharp and focused, aggressive, intelligent. Good powers of concentration | Calm, stoic; slow to learn but outstanding long-term memory |
| General disposition | Quick thinker, loves traveling and adventure; sensitive; creative or artistic | Clear-headed, practical, logical, goal-oriented, assertive | Calm, patient, loving, serious, passive |
| Dreams | Dreams a lot but doesn't remember them; scary dreams, violent dreams, dreams involving flying | Vivid, passionate or competitive dreams | Doesn't dream much; sentimental dreams or dreams involving water |
| Emotional tendency when imbalanced | Fearful, nervous, insecure, anxious, worried; blame themselves | Frustrated, angry, irritable, jealous; blame others | Depressed, complacent, overly sentimental or attached, stubborn |
| Speech style | Fast, variable tones; jumps from idea to idea; talks a lot | Focused, sharp voice; even or impatient tones; concise, logical; to the point | Often speaks slowly, sometimes in monotones, does not talk much |
| Movement style | Quick movements, walks impulsively, easily distracted | Goal-oriented, focused, direct, moves from point A to B | Slow, measured movements; prefers to move as little as possible |
| **YOUR TOTAL SCORE** | **VATA** ________ | **PITTA** ________ | **KAPHA** ________ |

These are the recommended diet and lifestyle guidelines for each dosha. Once you have determined your primary dosha, see below.

**AYURVEDIC RECOMMENDATIONS FOR EACH TYPE**

| RECOMMENDATIONS | VATA | PITTA | KAPHA |
|---|---|---|---|
| Dietary guidelines | Eat warm, nourishing foods with plenty of protein and fat. Don't skip meals; eat frequently at regular intervals on most days | Follow a cooling diet with plenty of raw foods; eat three main meals on most days | Eat light with modest portions and minimal amount of fat; avoid snacking and incorporate intermittent fasting regularly |
| Tastes to incorporate | Eat more sweet, sour, and salty tastes and reduce bitter, pungent, and astringent | Eat more sweet, bitter, and astringent tastes and reduce sour, salty, and pungent | Eat more bitter, pungent, and astringent tastes and reduce sweet, sour, and salty |
| Foods to incorporate | Hot foods, soups, stews, and hearty meals are encouraged. Sweet-tasting fruits like citrus and tropical fruits; root vegetables are good. Primarily eat cooked veggies | Sweet fruits like grapes, melons, and pomegranate; bitter vegetables and raw leafy greens are good. Consume ghee regularly, more so than other oils | Eat astringent fruits like apples, berries, and pears. Bitter and astringent vegetables like sprouts and artichokes are also good |
| Raw foods | Minimize raw foods or balance them with spices and oils e.g, ginger-sesame dressing | Include raw foods regularly such as salads and leafy green vegetables (which are energetically cooling) | Incorporate raw foods occasionally and balance them with warming spices |
| Meat | All types of meat are okay, ensure adequate protein in your diet; be cautious if eating vegetarian | Favor poultry and seafood over red meat; a vegetarian diet could work | A vegetarian diet may work for you; otherwise fish and seafood are best |

| RECOMMENDATIONS | VATA | PITTA | KAPHA |
|---|---|---|---|
| Avoidances | Avoid raw, cold, or frozen foods; avoid fried foods and dried fruits; minimize caffeine intake if you're sensitive to it | Reduce hot, spicy, or sour foods; avoid fried or greasy foods; avoid excessive alcohol; nighshade vegetables may be heating | Avoid dairy especially if it is mucus-producing for you, or opt for goat's milk products; avoid "emotional overeating"; caffeine is likely beneficial |
| Best spices | All spices in moderation are okay | Cumin, coriander, fennel, turmeric | Ginger, cardamom, cinnamon, turmeric |
| Lifestyle practices | Dress to stay warm and cover your head and ears; keep a regular daily routine and get plenty of sleep; seek out soothing, calming activities | Stay cool and avoid overheating; drink plenty of fluids; allow free time for rest and play; spend time in nature and near water | Keep warm, don't sleep too long and avoid naps; wake up early and perform brisk exercise; seek out stimulating new experiences; vary your routine |
| Exercise suggestions | Low-impact exercise, don't overdo it; yoga and meditation especially helpful | Moderate exercise, resist tendency to be overly competitive; team sports are preferable | High-intensity exercise recommended; some form of vigorous movement daily |
| Self-Abhyanga | Perform regular self-abhyanga with warm sesame oil | Perform self-abhyanga with coconut oil | Perform self-abhyanga either without oil or with almond oil |

## Strengthen Your Agni or Digestive Fire

The concept of *Agni*, or digestive fire, which determines our ability to digest, absorb, and assimilate our food, is fundamental to Ayurveda. Agni, which means "fire" in Sanskrit, refers broadly to your capacity to digest and process all experiences. Now we will focus on the physical Agni, which is a measure of your capacity to digest food. A healthy and strong Agni is indispensable for good health. If your Agni is weak, you will not be able to optimally extract nutrients and energy from the food you have taken, even if the food is of very high quality. Agni is correlated to some extent with stomach acid, digestive enzymes such as pancreatic enzymes, and bile from the gallbladder.

Signs of a healthy Agni include a healthy appetite, normal elimination, the absence of excessive gas or bloating, and normal energy levels. The strength of your Agni is a direct determinant of your capacity to effectively process raw foods, which are difficult to digest. This explains why certain people thrive on a raw-food diet (strong Agni), while other people actually may feel worse if they eat only raw foods.

If your Agni is weak, you will not break down your food properly, and that will lead to the production of *ama*, or toxins. Ama is a by-product of improperly digested food that in Ayurveda can accumulate in any part of the body, leading to inflammation and disease. It is believed that all disease begins with some imbalance in the gut that affects Agni, subsequently leading to the production of toxic ama, which is only later followed by the development of symptoms.

## Complexities of Ayurvedic Medicine

The science of Ayurveda is extremely complex, and for the purposes of this book, I have oversimplified it. You can imagine that three thousand years of practice has led to the development of a vast ocean of knowledge, of which I'm only presenting a small amount in this book.

Completing the questionnaire will give you an initial idea about your body type. However, an Ayurvedic practitioner will be able to come to a more accurate conclusion, based on history and physical examination including a detailed qualitative pulse exam (different from measuring heart rate) and tongue diagnosis. In addition, since doshas are always changing, your current state may be different from your original body type. It is also possible for more than one dosha to be imbalanced, in which case you would need to determine which one is the priority for treatment. As you can see, Ayurveda can become complex very quickly, so if you have any questions, please consult with your local Ayurvedic practitioner.

For the purposes of this book, try to determine what your original qualities and characteristics were, and aim to follow a regimen that will help restore your doshas to those of your constitution.

## Ayurvedic Therapeutics

There is an advanced understanding of various diseases and their therapies in Ayurveda. In order of potency, recommendations usually start with dietary change, followed by use of spices, and finally herbs and supplements. Mind-body techniques including meditation, breathing techniques, and yoga are commonly recommended as part of a treatment plan. We will discuss these in detail in Chapter 11.

There is also an intensive form of detoxification therapy known as panchakarma; while it is beyond the scope of this book, typically panchakarma is done in the inpatient setting in Ayurvedic hospitals or treatment centers. Patients, usually with more serious illnesses, may stay between two weeks to two months to receive the treatment, and I have seen some remarkable results with it.

## Ayurvedic Pathogenesis

There is a six-stage model in Ayurveda that explains how disease develops. Symptoms only appear at later stages, and the goal of Ayurveda is actually to detect imbalances and prevent disease before overt symptoms develop. In this way, Ayurveda is very focused on the root cause of disease and strongly emphasizes prevention. Therefore, Ayurveda is the original functional medicine, a modern specialty that assesses the function of different organ systems and attempts to uncover the root cause of illness. Ayurveda believes that all disease starts in the gut, at least to some degree, usually with weakening of the Agni.

1. Stage I—dosha imbalance and/or weakened Agni, leading to production of toxins (ama)
2. Stage II—imbalanced doshas build up in their respective organs
3. Stage III—doshas spread from their organs
4. Stage IV—imbalanced doshas and ama move to and localize at weak body tissues (dhatus), causing nonspecific symptoms
5. Stage V—early tissue damage occurs, major symptoms occur, leading to the development of a diagnosable disease
6. Stage VI—progressive disease, potentially with complications

Diseases at all stages are treatable, but the later the stage when treatment is begun, the more involved and time-consuming the therapy will be. The earlier that treatment is begun, the more likely the disease process can be fully reversed. If you are under the care of an Ayurvedic physician, the true measure of success would be catching imbalances at stage III or earlier, before symptoms have manifested, and addressing them before they progress any further.

## Eat All Six Tastes

In Ayurveda, food is described as having six different tastes. Most foods are a combination of two or more tastes; for example, coffee is considered both bitter and pungent. Some tastes are obvious—honey is considered sweet—but others are less intuitive, as ghee is also considered sweet.

It is ideal to consume foods from all six tastes in some form every day. If not possible, at least having as many different tastes as possible every day will help your diet to be more satiating and balanced.

The reason for this is that "taste" in Ayurveda has a sophisticated meaning that extends beyond the perceptions in your mouth. The six tastes each have different energetic and subtle effects on the doshas, with some increasing vata and others decreasing it, some having warming properties (thereby increasing pitta) and others cooling, and so forth. Therefore, ensuring that your diet has foods from all six different tastes is another strategy that helps promote the dosha balance, which in Ayurveda is indispensable for health.

Here is more information about foods in each taste category and the energetic properties and physiological effects of each taste:

## Table—The Six Different Tastes

| Taste | Examples of foods | Effects in the body |
|---|---|---|
| Sweet | Rice, whole grains, sweet potato, pumpkin, ghee; honey, molasses, and all natural sweeteners | Nourishing, rejuvenating, tonifying, strengthening |
| Sour | Lemon, tomato, citrus fruits, alcohol, yogurt, vinegar (apple cider vinegar is especially good), and all fermented foods | Stimulates saliva production, digestion, and appetite; aids in elimination |
| Salty | Salt of any type (Himalayan salt or sea salt recommended), seaweed, anchovies | Moisturizing, lubricating, clears obstructions, helps with fluid balance |
| Bitter | Leafy green vegetables, chocolate, coffee, turmeric, rhubarb, bitter melon, bitter gourd | Detoxifying, reducing inflammation, cooling, drying, balancing all other tastes |
| Pungent | Garlic, onion, ginger, chili, mustard, clove, black pepper, and most spices | Keeping the digestive fire strong, improving circulation, clearing mucus |
| Astringent | Brussels sprouts, asparagus, okra, cranberry, plantain, pomegranate, tea, chickpeas, lentils, sprouts of any type (e.g., alfalfa or clover) | Cleansing, purifying, removes excess moisture |

You can see from the table above how the different tastes have complementary properties and function like a system of checks and balances. Our modern diet typically has too much of the sweet and salty tastes. The tastes that are routinely underemphasized or missing in Western diets are the bitter and astringent tastes. Interestingly, these are the tastes that are most cooling in terms of energetic properties and would be especially helpful for reducing inflammation, which is considered a condition of excess heat or pitta in Ayurveda. Incorporating more of the pungent taste through spices can have a whole host of health benefits, as we discuss in Chapter 8.

The concept of six tastes is another unique lens that Ayurveda can offer to help ensure more balance in your diet. Again, it's important not to incorporate too much of any one taste, because excess use of a particular taste can also cause imbalances in the doshas. The key as in all things is moderation.

## The Paleovedic Approach

I have seen how people following a Paleo diet can inadvertently hurt themselves by not tailoring it to their Ayurvedic body type. Many people do not know that they need to customize Paleo for optimal results. Using Ayurveda to inform and customize a Paleo diet that is right for your constitution is the essence of the Paleovedic approach. Here are three examples that illustrate this.

## Case—Excess Vata

Jessica was a thirty-eight-year-old mother of two who came to see me for chronic constipation, fatigue, and anxiety. She was having small, hard bowel movements every three to four days and disabling anxiety that made it hard for her to function at work. She had switched to a Paleo-type diet a year before seeing me and initially felt more energy, but then she did not notice any improvement in symptoms. Her diet consisted of large salads daily for lunch and cold cuts or smoked salmon with vegetables for dinner. Her doctors had told her that drinking more water would help with her bowel movements, so she was drinking large quantities of iced water every day. She did not know why she was not feeling better despite avoiding all grains, eliminating gluten, and following a Paleo diet.

After getting her history and examining her, I determined that she had an excess of vata and a very weak Agni or digestive fire. Her daily salads and cold foods were in fact further increasing her vata and exacerbating her condition. A common symptom of elevated vata is anxiety, which was her most bothersome symptom. Her two water bottles per day filled with iced water were in fact depressing her Agni and further reducing her capacity to digest food effectively.

I had her change her diet to eliminate all raw foods such as salads and all cold foods. She began eating cooked vegetables, soups, and warm meat dishes instead of cold cuts. I told her to drink only warm or room temperature water and avoid ice. I instructed her to incorporate more spices into her cooking, such as turmeric, cumin, coriander, and ginger, to help stimulate her digestive fire and boost her metabolism. I encouraged her to use sesame oil, which is considered in Ayurveda to have medicinal properties for balancing vata dosha, in her everyday cooking.

Within two months, she reported that her chronic constipation had resolved. She was surprised to report that her anxiety had improved dramatically. Her energy, while not yet optimal, had increased to about 70 percent of normal. I reassured her that as she continued to balance her vata and strengthen her Agni, thereby improving her digestive capacity, her energy levels would return to normal.

## Case—Excess Pitta

Russell was a thirty-two-year-old male with severe ulcerative colitis, an autoimmune disease in which the body attacked the colon, leading to inflammation and loose stools. Despite being on the anti-inflammatory drug mesalamine, he still had elevated levels of C-reactive protein (CRP), a blood marker that indicated persistent inflammation. He was having eight to ten bowel movements per day with blood and mucus in his stools. He had been on a strict Paleo diet for six months, and his diet consisted of eggs, red meat, fermented dairy products, sauerkraut, and a limited number of vegetables.

After talking to him, I realized that he had excess pitta, which was manifesting as inflammation in his colon, bloody diarrhea, and a frequent sour taste in his mouth. I realized that the foods that he was eating were all very hot in terms of their qualities and properties. While meat, eggs, and dairy products are wonderful nutrient-dense foods, in his case they were actually not beneficial because of their heating properties.

I had him start a modified Paleovedic Detox without meat, eggs, or dairy products. For three weeks he consumed bitter greens such as arugula, spinach, and kale, which have very cooling energetic properties. I also encouraged him to eat *kitcheri* once a day, which he was open to doing even though it contained rice (which is not strictly Paleo by some definitions), because of its soothing effect on the gut. I encouraged him to liberally incorporate turmeric into his cooking. I suggested that he temporarily reduce consumption of sour foods such as sauerkraut because they can potentially aggravate pitta. Lastly, I suggested that he take a supplement containing *Boswellia serrata*, an herb that balances pitta and is often used to reduce inflammation.

At a three-month follow-up visit, he reported that his symptoms had improved by 80 percent. He was having two to three bowel movements per day, and there was no blood or mucus present in his stool. He was no longer experiencing the sour taste in his mouth. After continuing to work with me over the next year, we were able to wean him off the mesalamine and control his symptoms using diet and select supplements.

## Case—Excess Kapha

Rhonda was a fifty-four-year-old female who was struggling with obesity, fatigue, and a sluggish thyroid. Her TSH (thyroid stimulating hormone) had been hovering just outside the optimal range for many years. She had a strong aversion to taking medications and was opposed even to taking a natural form of thyroid hormone. She felt like she was too fatigued even to exercise, although she had been very active for most of her life. She was following a gluten-free Paleo diet with a lot of fruits and vegetables and loved dairy products of all kinds, including milk, cheese, and yogurt. She explained that she was from Wisconsin, where dairy farming is common, and that's why she loved drinking milk every day.

After talking with her, I determined that she had excess kapha as well as very low Agni. I had her follow a kapha-pacifying diet. Traditionally, Ayurveda recommends eliminating dairy products during such a diet. Even though it was very difficult for her, Rhonda stopped eating dairy products and started following the kapha meal plan. I also encouraged her to incorporate warming spices into her diet, such as ginger, turmeric, black pepper, and chili. Lastly, I suggested that she begin taking an herbal supplement called Guggulu, which is effective at reducing excess kapha and is traditionally used to support healthy thyroid function.

After three months, she was excited to report that she had lost fifteen pounds just from changing her diet. Her energy had improved to the point where she was able to start a regular exercise program. As she began exercising, her energy improved further, and she lost another ten pounds. After six months, we repeated her thyroid function tests and found that they had normalized.

## Conclusion

As you can see, there are many ways that Ayurveda can be used to help customize a Paleo diet that is right for your body type. Incorporating foods from all six different Ayurvedic tastes is also a helpful strategy to improve satiety and ensure a balance of different qualities and energies in your diet. Ayurveda has particular expertise in the realm of spices, which can be utilized to help take your health and nutrition to the next level; spices are discussed in the next chapter.

# CHAPTER 7

# THE KITCHEN PHARMACY—TWELVE POWERFUL HEALING SPICES

Ayurveda believes that spices, which are vastly underutilized by most of us, are truly medicinal. You likely have some spices in your kitchen but may not realize how impactful and therapeutic spices can be—and what a profound effect they can have on your health. In my experience, spices are not emphasized much within the Paleo community, and yet they are some the most nutrient-dense and antioxidant-rich foods on the planet. In fact, aside from organ meats, it is difficult to find a more concentrated food source of nutrients and phytochemicals than spices. Therefore, they are essential for people who value nutrient density and seek to prevent disease through natural means such as diet and lifestyle. The best part is that they make your food taste better at the same time!

Ayurveda considers spices to comprise an entire category of medicine, and this chapter is focused on twelve healing spices that I have selected after extensive research. I have chosen these spices based on several factors, primarily the potency of their health benefits, but also ease of use and availability. I call them "The Kitchen Pharmacy," and no kitchen should be without them. These twelve spices can be safely used by people of all body types and are mild enough for daily use.

Scientific research has uncovered profound healing effects from spices. The biochemistry and physiology behind these effects is now understood to be mediated by four main mechanisms—antioxidant, anti-inflammatory, blood sugar regulation, and digestive enhancement.

First, the spices listed here have unparalleled abilities to protect your body from oxidative stress through their rich array of antioxidants. Let's talk a little bit about why this is important.

Oxidative stress is one of the underlying mechanisms behind almost all major diseases and the aging process itself. Oxidative stress is the strain placed on our body as a result of internal processes like metabolism as well as external factors like environmental pollutants, radiation, and toxins.

Oxidative stress is caused by compounds known as free radicals, molecules that directly damage proteins, DNA, and other components of our cells.

Free radicals are also known as reactive oxygen species, or ROS. These molecules are produced in our body all the time as normal by-products of metabolism and other enzyme reactions. In the same way that an apple turns brown when exposed to air, you can think of a similar process of "rusting" occurring in our cells if they are exposed to excessive free radicals. The main benefit of antioxidants is that they protect our bodies from the damage caused by free radicals, and are therefore one of the main ways in which our body counteracts the effects of oxidative stress.

## How Do Antioxidants Work?

The old model was that your body runs low in antioxidants just like your car runs low on gas, and when you eat, you "fill up the tank" with antioxidants that protect against oxidative stress. The latest research is that this model is an oversimplification, and the reality is much more complex. In fact, some level of reactive oxygen species (ROS) may be beneficial for health; paradoxically, supplementation with antioxidants has been shown to be harmful.[1] How can we make sense of these findings?

Hormesis is the likely mechanism by which the antioxidants and phytochemicals in plants contribute to our health.[2] Hormesis is the process by which a stressor triggers a beneficial response. This may be easier to understand by looking at the example of exercise. During weightlifting, you are literally creating small tears in and thereby slightly injuring the muscles that you are working. However, with adequate nutrition and rest, the muscle will repair itself and be even stronger and healthier than it was before. Now, if you suddenly lift excess weight, you may cause a major injury that would not be easily repaired. Therefore, a small amount of stress makes you stronger, but too much stress is harmful. Like with all things, there is a healthy middle ground.

The antioxidants in fruits and vegetables activate some pathways of oxidative stress, but the result of this is a response by the body to trigger cellular repair pathways and stimulate intrinsic antioxidants. Therefore, the initial low-level stress and damage elicits a response in our body that makes it stronger and more resilient. This is how hormesis works. One oxidative stress pathway that is paradoxically activated by many dietary antioxidants is NF-E2-related factor 2, commonly known as Nrf2; antioxidants in our diet activate Nrf2, which leads to the creation of some reactive oxygen species in our cells, subsequently triggering an adaptive stress response.[3]

One study investigated the effects of consuming foods rich in flavonoids, which are well-known antioxidants. Consuming these foods did increase the body's antioxidant capacity, but not through significantly raising blood levels of flavonoids—rather, these foods triggered a hormetic response by which the body increased production of its endogenous antioxidants.[4]

The main point here is that eating foods that are rich in antioxidants, especially fruits, vegetables, and spices, is profoundly beneficial for health, partly because these foods "stress" our bodies in a beneficial way. However, taking antioxidants in supplement form is likely to be unhelpful or even harmful, because the hormesis process requires a delicate balance—and taking a few isolated antioxidants extracted from their whole foods will not have the same effect. In fact, studies have shown no benefit (and in some cases even possible harm) from taking antioxidant supplements—although antioxidant status in the body does matter. One study looked at people taking antioxidant supplements for over seven years and found no reduction in the risk of developing metabolic syndrome; however, having high blood levels of antioxidants did significantly decrease the risk of metabolic syndrome.[5] Therefore, having high levels of antioxidants as a result of a diet rich in fruits and vegetables is beneficial for health, but taking antioxidants in supplement form to try to boost your body levels may be counterproductive.

The second key property of spices is their anti-inflammatory effect. Many compounds in spices have the capacity to quiet inflammation, which is the underlying cause of most chronic disease. One of the key mechanisms by which many spices exert their beneficial effect is by blocking a compound known as Nuclear Factor-kappa B (NF-kB), which stimulates the expression of a broad array of inflammatory genes and is linked to multiple chronic diseases, including cancer, heart disease, Alzheimer's, and diabetes—phytochemicals from spices such as turmeric (curcumin), red pepper (capsaicin), cloves (eugenol), ginger (gingerol), cumin (anethol), fennel (anethol), rosemary (ursolic acid), and garlic (ajoene and others) have been shown to be effective at inhibiting the activation of NF-kB.[6]

Third, there is promising research suggesting that spices can help to maintain healthy blood sugar. In my clinical experience, optimal blood sugar regulation is fundamental to good health, so it's exciting to realize that spices can play a big role in maintaining glycemic and metabolic wellness.

Finally, spices are used in Ayurveda to maintain a healthy digestive tract and stimulate one's Agni, or digestive fire. Ayurveda believes that all disease starts in the gut, often with weakness in Agni, and that the main way to prevent disease is to maintain a strong Agni. Therefore, spices can be used as a fundamental tool for the maintenance of health and the prevention of illness through their beneficial effects on Agni.

## Primer on Research Terms

There is a remarkable amount of scientific literature on the therapeutic properties of spices. For each spice, I summarize some of the most important studies, focusing on clinical trials in humans and occasionally mentioning animal studies and laboratory research if they are significant.

The gold standard for medical research is the randomized double-blind placebo-controlled trial (RCT); whenever available, I discuss such studies. To explain the jargon, a "double-blind" study requires that both the participants and the researchers be "blinded"—neither group knows who is getting the active substance and who is getting the placebo, thus reducing bias. "Placebo-controlled" is when one group of patients gets the active compound and another group gets an inert substance or "placebo," so that all participants feel like they are taking something beneficial. This controls for the psychological effects of expectation and belief, which are quite powerful in their own right (I discuss the power of placebos in Chapter 11). Spices are part of an exciting frontier in medical research, and I hope we will see more well-designed studies in the years ahead.

I also review the safety profile of each spice, and discuss any contraindications or cautions for people with specific medical conditions. High doses of any spice could cause digestive upset, especially if you are not used to it. If this occurs, simply stop using the spice and reintroduce it in smaller doses to see if it is better tolerated. During pregnancy or breast-feeding, taking spices in a concentrated supplement form is contraindicated, except under the supervision of a licensed practitioner; using spices in a small amount for cooking is acceptable.

## Turmeric (*Curcuma longa*)

We begin with turmeric, the root of the plant *Curcuma longa*, which is my favorite spice and perhaps the one that is most rapidly gaining in popularity. I make sure to always find a way to consume turmeric every single day. One of the most well studied spices, turmeric has been analyzed in literally thousands of research studies. Turmeric has so many different positive physiological effects that it may be hard to believe that one spice could have such a plethora of health benefits.

However, the benefits of turmeric are indeed genuine and cannot be overstated. These effects are primarily a result of its potent antioxidant and anti-inflammatory properties, mediated by a dizzying array of biochemical mechanisms including effects on transcription factors, enzymes, cytokines, cell cycle proteins, receptors, and surface adhesion molecules.[7]

### Prescription Strength Anti-inflammatory

One of the key ingredients in turmeric, curcumin, has been shown to be effective at reducing inflammation through multiple mechanisms at the cellular level. As noted above, curcumin is effective at blocking NF-kB, a transcription factor that turns on the expression of genes related to inflammation and has been associated with various chronic diseases.

A number of animal and human studies have compared the efficacy of curcumin to prescription anti-inflammatories and found it to be equally effective, with fewer side effects. One RCT that compared turmeric against ibuprofen in patients with osteoarthritis of the knee found that 1,500 mg of a turmeric extract per day was as effective as 1,200 mg of ibuprofen in alleviating knee pain and stiffness and improving knee function, with fewer side effects such as abdominal discomfort.[8] A small study involving patients with rheumatoid arthritis (RA) found that curcumin was as effective as the prescription anti-inflammatory diclofenac at reducing pain and disease activity in RA.[9] Another RCT evaluated the use of curcumin to treat chronic anterior uveitis, a long-standing inflammatory disease of the eye, and found that curcumin was comparable in efficacy to conventional drug therapy.[10]

## King of Antioxidants

One of the key strengths of turmeric is its antioxidant potential. Its molecular structure enables it to function as an antioxidant and block free radicals directly. However, it also has the ability to stimulate the body's own production of antioxidants, which can potentially be even more powerful than antioxidants found in foods; turmeric has been shown to stimulate production of superoxide dismutase, glutathione reductase, and glutathione-s-transferase, three enzymes that are critical for the body's production of intrinsic antioxidants such as glutathione.[11]

## Cancer Fighter

In the area of cancer, a substantial body of research supports the idea that turmeric is effective against cancer. More than a thousand research studies have demonstrated that curcumin can fight cancer on many levels, both by inhibiting the development of cancer and preventing the growth and spread of cancer cells. It has exhibited powerful therapeutic effects against twenty-two different types of cancer, leading renowned cancer researcher Dr. Bharat Aggarwal to proclaim, "There is no other natural substance that has been found to possess this degree of anticancer power."[12]

## Protects the Heart

Turmeric is likely to be beneficial in preventing heart disease, the number one cause of death in the United States and worldwide. There are multiple different mechanisms by which turmeric supports healthy cardiovascular function, likely driven by its antioxidant and anti-inflammatory properties.[13] One of the mechanisms is a beneficial effect on the lining of blood vessels, known as the endothelium. One study conducted in postmenopausal women found that curcumin exerted a significant positive effect on endothelial function, which refers to how effectively the blood vessels are working.[14] Another RCT found that turmeric extract was better than placebo and equally effective as the prescription drug atorvastatin (Lipitor) at improving endothelial function and decreasing markers of inflammation and oxidative stress.[15] An RCT in high-risk patients who were undergoing coronary artery bypass graft (CABG) surgery found that curcumin was effective in reducing the incidence of post-surgery heart attacks in these patients by an impressive 65 percent.[16]

## Preserves Brain Function

Turmeric has neuroprotective effects that may make it a promising therapy for brain disorders such as Alzheimer's disease and Parkinson's disease. One of the characteristic features of Alzheimer's disease is the development of beta-amyloid plaques, deposits in the brain that affect memory and prevent normal cognitive functioning. In lab and animal studies, turmeric has been shown to be effective at reducing the deposition of beta-amyloid plaques in the brain and helping with clearance and removal of the plaques as well.[17] Turmeric has shown benefit in several animal models of Parkinson's disease, and curcumin has been shown to cross the blood-brain barrier.[18] In addition, certain brain disorders have been linked to declining levels of brain-derived neurotrophic factor (BDNF), a growth factor that stimulates neurons to multiply; turmeric has been shown to be effective at increasing brain levels of BDNF.[19] Some scientists suspect that the reason India has a relatively low incidence of Alzheimer's disease is because of the high rate of turmeric consumption.[20]

## Supports Detoxification

Turmeric is also traditionally used in Ayurveda as a "blood purifier"; it provides support for phase 2 liver detoxification pathways and can be used to help treat disorders of the liver and gallbladder. Interestingly, one study in patients with gallbladder disease found that daily supplemental curcumin was able to reduce the formation of gallstones and improve gallbladder health.[21]

## Beyond Curcumin

You may have noticed that most of the studies that I have referenced above referred to curcumin, one of the active ingredients in turmeric. Do all of the health benefits of turmeric derive from curcumin? You might think so, especially because a search for "curcumin" in PubMed, a government database of scientific research, brings up over six thousand citations. However, there is more to turmeric than just curcumin. Ayurveda always emphasizes using whole foods and prefers whole spices over their isolated constituents. In fact, research has looked at "curcumin-free turmeric" and found that it also has a variety of physiological effects including anti-inflammatory, anticancer, and blood sugar-lowering activity; other compounds in turmeric besides curcumin include "turmerin, turmerone, elemene, furanodiene, curdione, bisacurone, cyclocurcumin, calebin A, and germacrone."[22]

## Taking Turmeric as a Supplement

If you are seeking more systemic anti-inflammatory benefits from turmeric, it may be beneficial to take a turmeric supplement. The reason for this is that supplements can concentrate large quantities of the whole turmeric root, more than can be easily consumed as a powder. When turmeric is processed into an extract, the absorption and bioavailability are increased, and body tissues may be penetrated better for therapeutic effects. When choosing a turmeric supplement, it's ideal to select a product that has a good quality extract. One of the best forms of supplemental turmeric is a so-called "supercritical" formulation that uses carbon dioxide to create a full-spectrum extract from the whole root. This includes curcumin as well as other beneficial components of turmeric. Examples of brands that incorporate such a process include New Chapter Turmeric Force (capsule form) and Synchro Gold Turmeric Elixir (liquid form).

## Safety Profile

Turmeric has a good safety profile. Turmeric is about 2 percent curcumin by weight. Therefore, a tablespoon of turmeric, which weighs about 7,000 mg, contains about 140 mg of curcumin. Doses of up to 8,000 mg of curcumin (equivalent to 160 tablespoons of turmeric powder) per day have been shown to be safe for daily consumption for at least two months based on clinical trial data.[23] Obviously, it would be impossible to consume such a large amount of turmeric powder, which is why the powdered spice is very safe.

However, there are some cautions and contraindications for the use of turmeric supplements. Because of turmeric's blood-thinning properties, patients who are on blood-thinning medications such as warfarin (Coumadin) or high-dose nonsteroidal anti-inflammatory drugs (NSAIDs) should avoid turmeric supplements; for the same reason, it is recommended to discontinue turmeric supplements at least two weeks before any type of surgery. Because of its possible blood sugar–lowering effects, patients with diabetes who are on prescription medications should talk to their doctor before taking turmeric supplements. Patients with active liver disease, gallstones, or biliary obstruction should use caution with curcumin because of its potential to stimulate gallbladder contraction and bile secretion.[24] Pregnant and breast-feeding women should not take turmeric supplements because of lack of safety data but can safely use the spice in cooking.

## Incorporating Turmeric into Your Diet

With turmeric, it's a question of simply trying to consume as much as you can, in a variety of different forms. I recommend getting turmeric into your diet every day. Whenever possible, add some black pepper to accompany the turmeric, because this greatly increases the bioavailability and absorption of the turmeric—by 2,000 percent or 20 times in one study.[25]

Interestingly, many recipes in Indian cooking combine black pepper with turmeric, naturally achieving this synergy. Here are some ideas about how to incorporate turmeric into your diet (always try to add at least an eighth of a teaspoon of black pepper for each quarter teaspoon of turmeric you are adding):

1. Add some turmeric to the water in your rice cooker, and you will get a mildly flavored, beautiful yellow rice. Add about a quarter teaspoon of turmeric (and eighth teaspoon of black pepper) for every one cup of rice you are cooking.
2. When making creamy soups such as tomato soup, add turmeric to taste when you are simmering the soup on the stove.
3. When making scrambled eggs, add some turmeric into the mix before cooking the eggs.
4. For a simple beverage, mix a quarter teaspoon of turmeric in an eight-ounce glass of warm water. Stir well to dissolve. If you want to prepare a stronger herbal tea, add turmeric powder or turmeric root to boiling water and infuse for ten minutes; if you use turmeric root, discard the root before drinking. You may add raw organic honey to sweeten it and lemon juice for tartness. A variety of commercially available specialty beverages now contain turmeric. Look for these in your local health food store.
5. Incorporate turmeric into any marinade that you are using for any meat dish. It adds a great flavor to any meat or fish that you might be cooking.
6. Add turmeric to a morning smoothie. If you have a juicer, whole turmeric root may be used; alternatively, simply add some turmeric powder to the fruits and vegetables before blending.
7. Turmeric may be liberally added to any vegetables while sautéing, steaming, braising, or roasting them.
8. If you tolerate legumes, turmeric makes a great addition to lentils, chickpeas, or beans of any type. Turmeric also improves the digestibility of legumes, which is an added benefit.
9. Add some turmeric into your salad dressing, and shake well to disperse evenly before pouring it into your salad.
10. Turmeric can be mixed into yogurt dishes to provide a more savory yogurt, in contrast to sweeter yogurts with added fruit.

So-called "Golden Milk" is a wonderful beverage that incorporates turmeric and ginger. Traditionally made with regular milk, you can substitute any nondairy milk, like almond milk or coconut milk.

**Golden Milk**

Warm up some milk in a pan over medium heat. Add a quarter teaspoon each of turmeric and ginger, and an eighth teaspoon of black pepper, per eight ounces of milk. Stir well to mix the spices. Let the milk begin to simmer—small bubbles will form on the sides of the saucepan. Stir. Allow to heat for another minute or two. Then remove from heat and serve.

# Ginger (*Zingiber officinale*)

Ginger is the rhizome (technically the underground stem) of the ginger plant. It is used extensively in Ayurveda for its digestive benefits, anti-inflammatory properties, and energizing and stimulating effects. Like most spices, it is an outstanding source of antioxidants; its key phytochemicals include gingerols, paradols, shogaols, and gingerones.[26]

## Digestive Healer

Ginger is used traditionally in Ayurveda for digestive disorders such as indigestion, heartburn, and constipation. One common link between these three conditions is delayed emptying of the stomach and the resulting slowed movement of substances through the digestive tract, defined medically as decreased motility. If digested food does not leave the stomach properly and move through the intestines normally, it can predispose one to pain (indigestion or dyspepsia), reflux of acid (heartburn), and sluggish elimination (constipation). One ingenious double-blind placebo-controlled study used ultrasound imaging to show that ginger was effective at accelerating the emptying of the stomach and gently stimulating stomach contractions, thereby improving gastrointestinal motility.[27] This helps us understand why ginger may be helpful for digestive complaints.

One of the most well-established properties of ginger is its ability to reduce nausea and vomiting. Studies have proven that ginger is clearly effective for treating nausea from almost any cause; it provides symptomatic relief from seasickness, chemotherapy-associated nausea and vomiting, morning sickness during pregnancy, and postoperative nausea (a common complication after surgery).[28] The effects of ginger on gastric emptying and motility may be part of the explanation for its remarkable efficacy in treating nausea.

## Analgesic and Anti-inflammatory

Ginger also has a powerful capacity to reduce inflammation and joint pain. A number of studies have shown benefit for ginger in arthritis. One randomized controlled trial found that ginger powder was as effective as the prescription anti-inflammatory diclofenac at reducing pain and improving symptoms in patients with knee osteoarthritis over a twelve-week period.[29] Another randomized double-blind placebo-controlled trial found that ginger extract was better than placebo at reducing pain in patients with osteoarthritis of the knee.[30]

Ginger can also relieve other types of pain. An RCT from 2015 showed that ginger was able to reduce exercise-induced muscle pain; 2 g daily of ginger powder taken for eleven days significantly reduced pain compared to placebo, confirming ginger's analgesic effects for muscle pain in addition to joint pain.[31] This pain-relieving effect was also studied in women with primary dysmenorrhea, or painful menstrual periods. Another study showed that ginger was as effective at relieving menstrual pain as the pharmaceutical drugs ibuprofen and mefenamic acid when taken during the first three days of menstruation.[32]

## Anticancer Effects

One promising area of research is the potential role of ginger in prevention and treatment of cancer. A placebo-controlled study involving patients at increased risk of colon cancer found that a month of supplementing with ginger powder significantly improved specific biomarkers and favorably affected gene expression when compared to placebo.[33] Another study in an animal model of prostate cancer demonstrated that whole ginger extract inhibited the growth and progression of prostate cancer cells.[34] Lab studies in human ovarian cancer cells have found that a compound in ginger known as 6-gingerol is effective at reducing cell growth and modulating angiogenesis, the process by which tumors grow new blood vessels.[35]

## Improves Blood Sugar and Cholesterol

There is some evidence that ginger can be beneficial at improving metabolic status in patients with diabetes. For example, an RCT found that 1,600 mg of ginger per day was effective at lowering fasting blood sugar, improving insulin sensitivity, reducing the inflammatory marker CRP, and favorably affecting certain lipid parameters in patients with type 2 diabetes.[36] Another RCT in type 2 diabetics showed that 2 g per day of ginger powder lowered fasting blood sugar and hemoglobin A1c (a marker for blood sugar control over three months) and improved other heart disease risk markers after twelve weeks.[37]

## Fights Infections

Ginger is used traditionally in Ayurveda to fight infections and is especially helpful for sore throats, colds, and flus. One study showed that fresh ginger is active against a virus known as respiratory syncytial virus (RSV), a common cause of lung infections, especially in children.[38] Another study demonstrated the antibacterial activity of ginger, revealing that ginger was actually able to inhibit the growth of multidrug-resistant bacteria, which are clinically important bacteria that have become resistant to certain antibiotics.[39]

## Brain Tonic

Finally, ginger may have some benefit in terms of improving brain function. Research showed that ginger extract was able to enhance certain aspects of mental function, such as working memory and cognitive processing, in healthy middle-age women.[40]

You can see why I recommend daily consumption of ginger as part of your diet!

## Safety Profile

Ginger has an excellent safety profile. The most common mild side effect is gastrointestinal irritation. Because it is quite pungent, high doses of the spice may cause heartburn, diarrhea, or stomach upset.

Ginger as a spice is safe, but there are a few contraindications for use of the supplement. Patients on blood-thinning medications such as warfarin (Coumadin) or clopidogrel (Plavix) should avoid ginger because of possible herb-drug interactions. There is one case report in the literature of a patient on blood thinners who took ginger and had an herb-drug interaction causing nosebleeds (which resolved once the ginger was discontinued).[41]

As with all supplements, ginger extract should be stopped at least two weeks before any surgery because of the potential interactions with anesthesia medications and other unpredictable drug interactions.[42] Because of its beneficial effects on blood sugar, ginger should not be combined with prescription medications for diabetes except under the supervision of a physician. Ginger is often recommended as a treatment for symptoms experienced during pregnancy such as nausea, although I always recommend that pregnant women consult with their physicians before taking any dietary supplement.

Fresh ginger is considered the more potent form of the spice, but Ayurveda recommends liberal use of both fresh ginger and ginger powder. It can be used to add an aromatic note to any dish and can also be taken as a tea or an extract. Pickled ginger is another option that provides the additional benefits of a fermented food.

## Cinnamon (*Cinnamonum aromaticum*)

Cinnamon is actually the dried brown bark of the cinnamon tree. There are two main varieties of cinnamon, *Cinnamonum zeylanicum* (Ceylon cinnamon, also known as "true" cinnamon) and *Cinnamonum aromaticum* (Chinese cinnamon), which is also known as "cassia." Cinnamon cassia is less expensive and more widely available and fortunately has all of the health benefits revealed here.

Cinnamon is rich in antioxidants and polyphenols. A study comparing the antioxidant activity of twenty-six common spices found that cinnamon ranked second in antioxidant potency (behind only clove).[43] Some of the beneficial phytochemicals in cinnamon include cinnamaldehydes, flavonoids, and volatile oils.[44]

## Lowers Cholesterol and Blood Sugar

Cinnamon shows exceptional promise for treating metabolic issues like elevated blood sugar and abnormal lipids. One recent meta-analysis that reviewed ten randomized controlled trials found that "consumption of cinnamon is associated with a statistically significant decrease in levels of fasting plasma glucose, total cholesterol, LDL, and triglyceride levels, and an increase in HDL levels."[45] Several possible mechanisms have been proposed for these glycemic benefits, such as improvement of insulin sensitivity and glucose uptake.

## Reduces Inflammation

Cinnamon also has beneficial blood-thinning properties, which are mediated by its ability to prevent blood components known as platelets from clumping together excessively; this effect is partially due to the anti-inflammatory effects of cinnamon, suggesting that it may be helpful in reducing chronic inflammation.[46] There are several compounds that have been isolated from cinnamon that have shown anti-inflammatory properties; these include gnaphalin, hesperidin, hibifolin, hypolaetin, oroxindin, and quercetin.[47]

All the above properties, such as thinning the blood, reducing inflammation, and improving blood sugar and cholesterol parameters, suggest that cinnamon may be beneficial for protecting the heart and keeping the cardiovascular system healthy. Animal studies have shown benefit for cinnamon in heart disease; the effects may be mediated by phytochemicals in cinnamon such as cinnamic aldehyde, cinnamophilin, and cinnamic acid.[48]

## Helping PCOS

Cinnamon also shows promise in helping to treat polycystic ovarian syndrome (PCOS), the most common hormone imbalance in women of reproductive age and one of the most common causes of female infertility. A pilot study conducted in women with PCOS demonstrated that a daily cinnamon extract taken for eight weeks was effective in lowering blood sugar and reducing insulin resistance, one of the primary metabolic abnormalities in PCOS.[49]

## Natural Antimicrobial

Traditionally used in Ayurveda for its antimicrobial properties, cinnamon has been shown to have antibacterial and antifungal effects in lab studies as well. One study demonstrated that cinnamon was effective in inhibiting the growth of a pathogenic fungus known as *Candida albicans*.[50] Another study conducted by food scientists found that the essential oil of cinnamon was able to inhibit the growth of five out of six bacteria that are often involved in food spoilage.[51]

## Safety Profile

Cinnamon has a good safety profile when used in small quantities as a spice. However, there is a risk in consuming large quantities of cinnamon cassia over time, because of a compound known as coumarin. Occurring naturally in many plants including cinnamon cassia, coumarin is safe and poses no risk at doses of up to 0.1 mg per kilogram of body weight per day, according to a German government agency.[52] The European Union actually regulates the amount of coumarin in foods such as baked goods that contain cinnamon. In fact, there was a minor scandal in 2006 in Germany when Christmas cinnamon cookies were found to exceed allowable levels of coumarin—it was later determined that people would have to eat more than fifteen cinnamon cookies per day to exceed safe levels, so they were just advised to enjoy the cookies in moderation (no adverse reactions were actually reported).[53]

Up to one teaspoon per day of cinnamon cassia is safe for daily consumption; I would not exceed this amount for long periods of time, except under the supervision of a physician. Interestingly, coumarin is only present in cinnamon cassia and is not found in Ceylon cinnamon (*Cinnamonum zeylanicum*). Therefore, if you would like to use higher doses of cinnamon for additional therapeutic effects, I would recommend Ceylon cinnamon (also known as "true" cinnamon). While most grocery stores sell cinnamon cassia, Ceylon cinnamon is available in specialty foods stores and online in powder, stick, and supplement forms. Cinnamon is safe to consume as a spice during pregnancy, but do not take cinnamon supplements during pregnancy or breast-feeding because of unknown possible adverse effects.

## Practical Tips

Cinnamon can be incorporated into your diet in many ways, in both sweet and savory dishes. It works well as an addition to smoothies. I usually add a teaspoon of cinnamon powder whenever I make a morning smoothie.

**Dr. Akil's Super-Spice Morning Smoothie**

8 ounces of filtered water

3 ounces of blueberries or strawberries

1 scoop organic grass-fed whey protein

1 tablespoon of raw cacao powder

1 tablespoon of coconut oil

1 tablespoon of flaxseeds or chia seeds

¼ teaspoon of cinnamon powder

¼ teaspoon of cardamom powder

⅛ teaspoon of turmeric powder

⅛ teaspoon of black pepper

liquid stevia extract or raw honey to taste

# Cumin (*Cuminum cyminum*)

Cumin, commonly known as *jeera*, is a ubiquitous ingredient in Indian curries but also appears often in Middle Eastern, Mexican, and African dishes. It is a small, oblong, brownish seed that resembles the more familiar caraway seed. It has a distinct flavor because it contains cuminaldehyde, a compound with remarkable medicinal qualities; it is also rich in antioxidants known as flavonoids.[54] Cumin is nutrient-dense, is an excellent source of iron, and is loaded with minerals such as manganese, potassium, calcium, magnesium, and phosphorus.

## Stimulates Digestion

Cumin's primary use in Ayurveda is to stimulate and strengthen digestion, which is corroborated by research showing that cumin can stimulate the production of pancreatic enzymes that are vital to proper digestion.[55] Cumin is one of the few Ayurvedic spices (along with fennel and coriander) that help strengthen the digestive fire without aggravating pitta. Therefore, it can be used safely by people of all body types.

## Regulates Blood Sugar

Cumin shows promise in balancing blood sugar. A number of studies in animal models of diabetes found that cumin was comparable in effectiveness to certain prescription medications in lowering blood sugar and treating diabetes.[56] Cumin may reduce the production in diabetics of harmful compounds known as advanced glycation end products, or AGEs.[57]

## Improves Cholesterol

Like most spices that can help lower blood sugar, cumin also seems to be helpful in normalizing cholesterol. It is increasingly recognized that oxidized LDL cholesterol particles play a role in the development of heart disease. In a study with thirty-nine healthy people, cumin extract was shown to be effective at reducing levels of oxidized LDL and increasing the levels of enzymes that protect against oxidation of LDL and help clear cholesterol plaques from blood vessels.[58]

## Protects against Cancer

Cumin shows significant cancer-fighting potential. Animal studies have shown that cumin could reduce the risk of cervical, stomach, and liver cancer as well as prevent the occurrence of colon cancer in rats fed cancer-causing substances.[59]

## Prevents Bone Loss

Cumin may be beneficial for bone health and shows potential in the treatment of osteoporosis, a degenerative condition in which the bones become weak and brittle, predisposing one to fractures. In an animal model of osteoporosis, cumin extract was comparable to the prescription hormone estradiol in preventing bone loss; it was able to increase bone density and bone strength without having the side effects of estradiol such as weight gain and excessive endometrial stimulation.[60]

### Kills Bad Bacteria

Cumin was traditionally used in India as part of spice blends to help preserve foods; it likely worked by inhibiting the growth of bacteria that cause food spoilage. Studies have shown that cumin essential oil has antibacterial activity against a variety of different kinds of bacteria.[61]

### Practical Tips

Cumin seeds work well if they are dry roasted in a small quantity of oil or ghee at the beginning of cooking. Cumin seed powder is fragrant and adds a wonderful aromatic flavor to meat, vegetable, or bean dishes. Cumin has an excellent safety profile with no major adverse reactions reported in the literature.

## Black Cumin (*Nigella sativa*)

While black cumin (no relationship to cumin) is neither easy to find nor routinely used in Indian cooking, it is a spice that has tremendous healing potential. For those willing to go to the extra mile to obtain it, the rewards in terms of health benefits are significant. Black cumin is a small, black seed that has the sheen of obsidian—it looks nothing like cumin because it comes from a different botanical family.

### Medicinal Cornucopia

Black cumin is a veritable gold mine of medicinal properties—research shows potential health benefits in a long list of medical problems, including heart disease, cancer, asthma, allergies, autoimmune disease, inflammatory bowel disease, eczema, high blood pressure, multiple sclerosis, epilepsy, stomach ulcers, and other conditions. There are more than a hundred different compounds that have been identified so far in black cumin, including amino acids; essential fatty acids; vitamins; minerals including calcium, iron, and potassium; and a unique bionutrient called thymoquinone, which is not found in any other plant.[62] In clinical studies, *Nigella sativa* (the botanical name is commonly used interchangeably with "black cumin") has shown anti-inflammatory, anticancer, pain-relieving, immune-boosting, and fever-reducing properties.[63]

## Antioxidant Booster

Black cumin has been shown to be not only rich in antioxidants but also to have the capacity to strengthen the body's own antioxidant defense systems by modulating enzymes relating to glutathione, the master antioxidant in the body.[64]

## Lowers Blood Pressure

*Nigella sativa* is used traditionally as a remedy for hypertension. It was shown in a randomized, double-blind placebo-controlled trial to lower both systolic and diastolic blood pressure in healthy individuals after two months of daily consumption.[65]

## Normalizes Blood Sugar

Black cumin shows significant potential as an agent that can help maintain healthy blood sugar. In a study looking at patients with type 2 diabetes, taking 2 g of black cumin daily was shown to reduce fasting blood sugar and hemoglobin A1c (a measure of blood glucose control over three months) as well as lower insulin resistance and improve the activity of cells in the pancreas.[66] These were patients who are already taking oral diabetes drugs, suggesting that black cumin can be a good adjunctive therapy even for patients on prescription medications.

## Improves Lipid Profiles

The seeds also show promise in treating hyperlipidemia. A randomized placebo-controlled clinical trial with *Nigella sativa* powder showed a significant decrease in total and LDL cholesterol and a remarkable 16 percent drop in triglycerides after two months of daily consumption.[67] In a randomized placebo-controlled trial with postmenopausal women, black cumin was shown to have a favorable impact on cholesterol levels, increasing beneficial HDL and lowering potentially harmful LDL when compared to a placebo.[68]

## Reduces Inflammation

The ability of *Nigella sativa* to reduce inflammation and modulate the immune system was put to the test in a study with patients suffering from rheumatoid arthritis. *Nigella sativa* oil was able to effectively reduce pain, swelling, and morning stiffness when compared to a placebo after daily use for one month.[69]

## Natural Antimicrobial

Black cumin is traditionally used in Ayurveda for its antimicrobial activity. These properties, including antiparasitic and antifungal effects, have been documented in multiple studies.[70]

## Supports Fertility

Because *Nigella sativa* has been traditionally used to help treat infertility, studies have investigated its effect on men with unexplained male infertility. One RCT found that *Nigella sativa* oil was able to improve sperm count, morphology, and motility as well as semen volume in men with fertility problems after two months of daily administration.[71]

## Safety Profile

Black cumin is a very safe compound; the only adverse reactions reported in the literature are two cases of contact dermatitis when people experienced skin irritation from using *Nigella sativa* oil topically.[72] The whole seed is safe to consume as a spice during pregnancy, but the supplement form should be avoided in pregnancy because animal studies suggest that *Nigella sativa* may inhibit or prevent uterine contractions.[73]

## Practical Tips

To find black cumin, you have to venture beyond the traditional supermarket to specialty stores, health food stores, or Indian markets, where it is often sold under the name *Nigella sativa* or *kolonji*. It is also available online. The seeds can be used whole and do not have to be ground into powder. They have a mild peppery taste and add an aromatic flavor to recipes; they can be liberally added to meat, vegetable, and bean dishes and can be used in sauces and soups.

## Fenugreek (*Trigonella foenum-graecum*)

Fenugreek, also known as *methi*, is a beloved spice in most Indian kitchens, with both the seeds and the leaves being used. It is revered in Ayurveda for its beneficial effects on a variety of health conditions. Research on fenugreek has been extensive. Its therapeutic constituents include phytochemicals known as saponins, the unusual amino acid 4-hydroxyisoleucine, a unique alkaloid called trigonelline, and a high fiber content.[74]

### Metabolic Powerhouse

Fenugreek is one of the most powerful spices for addressing metabolic issues such as problems with blood sugar and cholesterol. In fact, over a hundred studies—mostly in animals with experimentally induced diabetes but also in human trials—demonstrate fenugreek's power to help with blood sugar regulation and improve other metabolic imbalances such as high total cholesterol, high triglycerides, and low beneficial HDL cholesterol.[75]

### Lowers Blood Sugar

One meta-analysis that reviewed ten clinical studies on fenugreek concluded that fenugreek, when taken in adequate doses of at least 5 g per day, can have a beneficial effect on fasting blood sugar, postprandial (after meals) blood sugar, and hemoglobin A1c (a three-month measure of blood sugar used to assess long-term glycemic control).[76] Another innovative study involving bread made from ground fenugreek seeds showed that "fenugreek bread" was effective at reducing insulin resistance, suggesting that there are multiple ways to incorporate fenugreek into one's diet.[77]

### Improves Cholesterol and Triglycerides

In one study with type 2 diabetics, fenugreek powder was shown to be beneficial in reducing blood sugar and favorably affecting triglycerides and cholesterol.[78] Another double-blind placebo-controlled study also involving type 2 diabetics found that fenugreek seed extract improved blood sugar, decreased insulin resistance, reduced triglycerides, and increased beneficial HDL cholesterol.[79]

## Traditional Use

Fenugreek is used traditionally in Ayurveda as a galactagogue, a substance that stimulates breast milk production in postpartum women, although there are no good-quality research studies that have investigated this property.

## Safety Profile

Fenugreek has a good safety profile, with the most common side effects reported being mild gastrointestinal upset and rarely a maple syrup–like odor in the urine (a by-product of fenugreek metabolism); because of possible cross-reactivity, patients with allergies to peanuts, chickpeas, or coriander should avoid fenugreek.[80] In addition, pregnant women should avoid fenugreek because a miscarriage or early labor could be triggered by the phytoestrogens in the spice. For the same reason, women with estrogen-dependent breast or ovarian cancer should avoid fenugreek.

## Practical Tips

Fenugreek is available in both seed and powder form. I prefer the powder form because a pinch can be easily added to many dishes while cooking; a little bit goes a long way. The seeds are difficult to chew and should always be cooked well before eating. Fenugreek adds a savory note to most dishes and can be used in curries, meats, and sautéed vegetables.

# Clove (*Eugenia caryophyllus*)

Cloves are the dried, unopened flower buds of the clove tree; they resemble small nails, and in fact their name is derived from the Latin word for nail, clavus. They are rich sources of vitamin K, fiber, and minerals, including magnesium, iron, calcium, and manganese.[81]

## Best in Class Antioxidant

Clove is a simple, unassuming spice that is an antioxidant superpower. In a study that measured antioxidant capacity of twenty-four common spices based on their ability to prevent formation of advanced glycation end products, or AGEs (harmful by-products of high blood sugars), clove was the compound that was ranked number one.[82] Clove was also the clear winner in another study comparing the antioxidant potency of twenty-six spice extracts using a different methodology.[83]

## Reduces Inflammation

Clove has powerful anti-inflammatory properties; in one study, it was able to reduce blood levels of inflammatory markers after just seven days in volunteers who consumed a small amount of clove daily.[84] One good thing about this study is that it attempted to replicate typical daily consumption of spices and not what one would get from taking a concentrated supplement; this supports the idea that regular consumption of small quantities of spices, as is usually done in cooking, has measurable therapeutic effects. It also demonstrated benefit after only seven days of consumption, suggesting that spices can effect measurable changes rather quickly.

## Supports Wound Healing

This anti-inflammatory power is likely responsible for clove's beneficial effects in a clinical study on patients with anal fissures. An embarrassing but unfortunately common problem, anal fissures are difficult to treat, and surgical treatment carries a significant risk of partial or complete incontinence. One study of topical clove oil cream found that it was effective at healing anal fissures in 60 percent of patients after six weeks, compared to standard nonsurgical treatment, which healed only 12 percent of patients.[85]

## Relieves Pain

Clove is remarkably effective as a topical anesthetic and is used in dentistry for its anesthetic and analgesic properties; it is thought that eugenol is the phytochemical in clove that is responsible for its anesthetic effects.[86]

### Inhibits Bacteria and Fungi

Clove is traditionally used in Ayurveda for its antimicrobial effects, especially against bacterial and parasitic infections. Research has confirmed that clove oil is effective at inhibiting the growth of foodborne pathogens and certain bacteria.[87] Eugenol from clove oil also seems to have antifungal activity, and even the likely mechanism by which it inhibits fungal growth has been determined.[88]

### Practical Tips

Whenever possible, purchase whole cloves, as clove powder tends to lose its potency rather quickly. Clove may be used in sweet dishes such as pumpkin pie and also in savory dishes like curries, chili, and beans. Clove has an excellent safety profile, and adverse reactions have not been reported.

## Fennel (*Foeniculum vulgare*)

Fennel is one of the most highly valued spices in the Ayurvedic pharmacopeia, commonly used to strengthen digestion, reduce inflammation, and clear toxins. Its pleasant, fruity aroma inspires its extensive use in Indian dishes. Its digestive properties are the reason you commonly find a bowl of fennel seeds near the exit in an Indian restaurant.

### Powerful Antioxidant

Fennel's antioxidant portfolio includes rutin, quercetin, and kaempferol glycosides, but perhaps its key phytonutrient is a compound called anethole, which in animal studies has been consistently shown to reduce inflammation and prevent cancer, likely by modulating an intracellular signaling pathway called tumor necrosis factor alpha.[89] It has been found to have very potent antioxidant properties, even greater than the well-known antioxidant vitamin E.[90]

### Improves Digestion

One randomized placebo-controlled trial of fennel seed oil in infants with colic, a common digestive disorder, found that fennel seed oil was remarkably effective at reducing pain and improving digestion when compared to a placebo.[91] Fennel is highly prized in Ayurveda because of its ability to stimulate and strengthen the digestive fire (or Agni) without excessively heating the body and potentially aggravating pitta.

### Pain Reliever

Another study looked at the effects of fennel in reducing menstrual-related pain in young women. It found that an extract of fennel was equally effective as an over-the-counter nonsteroidal anti-inflammatory drug (NSAID) at reducing menstrual pain.[92]

### Cancer Fighter

Fennel may have anticancer properties as well. In animal models of skin cancer and stomach cancer, fennel was found to be protective against the development of cancer.[93]

### Practical Tips

In cooking, the entire fennel plant—including bulb, stalk, leaves, and seeds—can be used. In Ayurveda, the seeds are traditionally used. Fennel seeds work well when they are dry roasted in a small amount of coconut oil or ghee at the beginning of a recipe; this is the way they are traditionally used in Indian cooking. The seeds may also be liberally sprinkled in soups, curries, and a variety of meat and vegetable dishes. Fennel has an excellent safety profile, and there are no contraindications to its use.

## Coriander (*Coriandrum sativum*)

Coriander is one of the most ancient culinary herbs and is used extensively in India but also in Europe, Asia, Latin America, and the Middle East. Its name originates from the Greek *koriannon*, meaning "bug," a reference to the smell of the leaves. [94] The leaves of the coriander plant are commonly known as cilantro, which you are likely to be familiar with because of its widespread availability. Although studies have not been done in this area, cilantro extract is often used by herbalists to help treat excess body levels of heavy metals such as mercury and lead.

The ripened seeds of the plant, strongly aromatic with a slightly bitter edge, are used frequently in Indian cooking. Coriander seeds are either spherical or egg-shaped and usually yellowish-brown with a longitudinal ridge.

## Rich in Antioxidants

Coriander has potent antioxidant activity and is rich in phytochemicals, including phenolics, tannins, and flavonoids; much like turmeric, it seems to be able to induce enzymes that help the body to make its own powerful antioxidants, such as glutathione.[95] Coriander was shown to protect human skin cells from the effects of toxin-induced damage by counteracting effects of oxidative stress and activating proteins involved in cellular repair.[96]

## Improves Digestion

Coriander is especially helpful for digestive complaints. According to Ayurveda, it can be used to help relieve gas and discomfort, reduce bloating, and strengthen the digestive fire. This was corroborated in one research study that evaluated Carmint, an herbal formula that contains coriander, spearmint, and another plant known as lemon balm. In a randomized placebo-controlled trial, Carmint was shown to be superior to placebo at reducing the severity and frequency of abdominal pain and reducing abdominal bloating in patients with irritable bowel syndrome.[97]

In fact, the German Commission E, a government agency that makes recommendations about herbal medicines, declared that coriander is "safe and effective for the treatment of digestive complaints, loss of appetite, bloating, flatulence, and cramp-like stomach upsets."[98]

## Normalizes Blood Sugar and Cholesterol

Ayurvedic medicine often utilizes coriander when metabolic support for blood sugar and cholesterol is needed. A number of animal studies suggest that coriander may help normalize blood sugar in cases of diabetes.[99] One study demonstrated blood sugar–lowering effects of coriander extract that are equivalent to the prescription drug glibenclamide; coriander also had positive metabolic effects such as favorably affecting cholesterol and triglyceride numbers.[100] Another study confirmed that coriander seeds were able to increase levels of beneficial HDL cholesterol and lower levels of potentially harmful LDL cholesterol.[101]

## Fights Infections

Coriander has significant antimicrobial activity and may be used in Ayurveda as part of a treatment protocol to fight infections. Coriander essential oil was shown to be topically effective at inhibiting the growth of common skin bacteria.[102] Coriander has also demonstrated antifungal activity in laboratory studies; this was confirmed when coriander essential oil was shown to be an effective treatment against athlete's foot, a common toe fungus.[103]

## Safety Profile

Coriander has an excellent safety profile, and few adverse effects have been reported. There have been a few case reports of allergic anaphylactic reactions to cilantro.[104] If you have any type of allergic reaction to cilantro, you should avoid coriander because it is derived from the same plant. There was a report of contamination of coriander powder with chemicals known as phthalates, which are toxic compounds derived from plastics.[105] It is not clear how the coriander became contaminated with phthalates, but with most spices in general and coriander in particular, I recommend trying to purchase the certified organic form to reduce the possibility of adulteration.

## Practical Tips

Whole seeds are easy to crush and last for two years, but coriander powder is also widely available. As with all spices, purchase coriander powder in small quantities because the volatile oils tend to lose their potency more quickly once the spice has been ground. Coriander is one of the few Ayurvedic spices that help stimulate digestion and strengthen the digestive fire without aggravating pitta. Therefore, it can be used safely by people of all body types.

My wife, who uses spices a great deal, tells me that coriander is the one powdered spice that can be added liberally to a dish without overwhelming or overpowering it. In fact, if any other spice has been added to excess, adding coriander powder will help to balance the taste. Coriander seeds make a tasty addition to soups and broths, and coriander powder can be liberally added to meat dishes, curries, sautéed vegetables, and even pancake mix. The coriander seeds can also be placed in a pepper mill and sprinkled on top of cooked dishes at the table.

## Allspice (*Pimenta dioica*)

Allspice, also known as Jamaican pepper, is the dry unripe fruit of the *Pimenta dioica* tree. It is so named because it has flavor notes and aromas that remind one of many different spices, such as cloves, nutmeg, and cinnamon. Allspice is extremely popular in South America and the West Indies, where it is most famous as a key ingredient in jerk marinades for meat dishes. In fact, it was discovered by Christopher Columbus in Jamaica, who mistakenly thought that he had found black peppercorns, which were traded as currency during that time.[106] It is rather hot and peppery and in terms of medicinal properties is similar to clove.

### Potent Antioxidant

Allspice is rich in antioxidants, containing at least twenty-five active antioxidant compounds including quercetin, eugenol, and ellagic acid; it also has antiviral and antibacterial qualities to fight infections and analgesic properties that can help with pain relief.[107] In a study comparing the antioxidant potency of common herbs, allspice ranked second behind only clove.[108]

### Traditional Use

Allspice is used as a folk remedy to help relieve indigestion and also balance the menstrual cycle. Researchers studying traditional remedies for menopause found that allspice had the capacity to modulate genes involved in estrogen, thus providing a plausible mechanism and explanation for why allspice is used to treat menopausal symptoms in South America.[109]

## Cancer Fighter

One interesting animal study showed anticancer effects in prostate cancer; one particular compound called ericifolin, which was isolated from allspice berries, is believed to be responsible for this antitumor effect.[110] Studies in humans with prostate cancer would be interesting.

## Regulates Blood Pressure

Animal studies suggest a possible blood pressure–lowering effect thought to be mediated by relaxation of the nervous system and improvement of blood flow through the blood vessels.[111]

## Practical Tips

To maintain the potency of allspice, it's best to purchase the whole dried berries rather than the ground powder. The spice is extremely versatile. It is easily crushed in a mortar or by hand before adding to dishes. It can be used in stews, soups, dishes with legumes, curries, and meat loaf, and also blends well in sweet dishes such as pies, puddings, and cakes.[112] It is traditionally used in South America to spice up chocolate. Allspice has an excellent safety profile.

# Curry Leaf (*Murraya koenigii*)

Curry leaf (not to be confused with curry powder, which is a blend of different spices) is a small, green, leafy plant native to South Asia that is used extensively in Indian cooking. In Ayurvedic medicine, it is traditionally used to help with diabetes, heart disease, and chronic inflammation.

## Rich in Antioxidants

Curry leaf is loaded with antioxidants, more so than many other green leafy plants, due to a unique set of antioxidants, including carbazole alkaloids, triterpenoids, and flavonoids.[113] Curry leaf also contains other antioxidants, including quercetin, epicatechin, rutin, naringin, and myricetin.

## Regulates Blood Sugar

While human studies are limited, animal studies with curry leaf have shown promise for a variety of conditions. Certain animal studies suggest that curry leaves may have the capacity to regulate blood sugar in diabetes.[114] One study showed that curry leaf had a protective effect against diabetes-induced kidney damage.[115]

## Reduces Inflammation

One study demonstrated that curry leaf extract had an equivalent anti-inflammatory effect to a pharmaceutical drug called diclofenac.[116]

## Supports Cognitive Function

Curry leaf extract was shown to have cholesterol-lowering properties and the capacity to help with memory loss and cognitive impairment.[117]

## Cancer Fighter

Possibly as a result of their potent antioxidants, extracts of curry leaf were shown to have anticancer activity in lab studies using human cancer cells.[118] Curry leaf extract was also shown to reduce the number of tumors in animals with chemically induced colon cancer.[119]

## Practical Tips

Curry leaf is available in most Indian markets and also available online. For maximum potency, it's best to use fresh curry leaves that are still attached to the stem. They will last for about a week in the refrigerator and can be stored in the freezer, where they will keep for about three months. They might turn a dark, almost black color in the freezer, but this does not affect their flavor adversely. They can be used frozen and do not have to be thawed for cooking.

In Indian cooking, curry leaf is often added whole but picked out during the process of eating and usually not consumed with the dish. While many of the nutrients from curry leaf do enter into the dish, for maximum benefit, consume the whole curry leaf after cooking. Another alternative that works well is to finely chop or purée curry leaf together with other spices so that it can be consumed more easily. Curry leaf is safe, and adverse reactions have not been reported.

## Ajwain (*Trachyspermum ammi, Carum copticum*)

Ajwain, also known as ajowan or carom, is a spice that is not well-known in the West but is used extensively in India both in cooking and in traditional medicine, where the seeds, flowers, oils, and extracts are utilized. Ajwain contains a number of beneficial phytochemicals, including glucosides, saponins, carvacrol, volatile oils (thymol), terpiene, paracymene, and beta-pinene; it is also nutrient-dense and an excellent source of fiber, vitamin $B_3$ (niacin), and minerals including calcium, phosphorus, and iron.[120] The high concentration of the aromatic compound thymol in ajwain often reminds people of thyme, which is also rich in thymol.

### Traditional Use

Ayurveda commonly uses ajwain for colds, viral infections, asthma, kidney stones, and digestive disorders, including heartburn, gas, bloating, and indigestion. Often in Indian restaurants, you will see a bowl near the door containing a mixture of fennel seeds and ajwain, which are chewed after the meal to ensure healthy digestion.

### Supports Respiratory Health

Ayurveda employs ajwain to help treat respiratory conditions such as asthma, which typically involves pulmonary airway constriction and inflammation that makes it difficult to breathe. A study comparing ajwain extract to the prescription asthma medication theophylline found that the ajwain extract was almost as effective at opening up the airways and helping patients to breathe as the prescription drug.[121] One animal study assessing a different pulmonary condition found that ajwain extract was, in fact, more effective than the prescription drug codeine at relieving cough.[122]

## Lowers Blood Pressure

In animal models of high blood pressure, ajwain extract was shown to be effective at lowering blood pressure and slowing the heart rate.[123] In another study, ajwain was shown to be as effective as the prescription drug verapamil, which works by blocking calcium channels, at lowering high blood pressure.[124] The same study demonstrated that ajwain extract had liver-protective properties and could prevent signs of liver damage typically observed after exposure to certain toxins.

## Improves Digestion

A number of animal studies have demonstrated digestive benefits of ajwain, including treatment of peptic ulcer, improved activity of digestive enzymes, and reduction in stomach discomfort and pain.[125]

## Fights Infections

Ajwain is traditionally used in Ayurveda to combat infections such as viral, bacterial, and parasitic diseases. Its antibacterial activity was confirmed in a study that evaluated various essential oils against potentially pathogenic intestinal bacteria and fungi—ajwain seed essential oil was powerfully effective in selectively inhibiting the growth of harmful gut microbes that could potentially cause dysbiosis (such as clostridium bacteria and the yeast candida), without having a negative impact on beneficial bacteria.[126]

## Practical Tips

Ajwain has an excellent safety profile, and adverse reactions have not been reported in the literature. It can be consumed in either whole seed or powder form. It can be found commonly in Indian grocery stores and is available online. It is best to cook the seeds first, preferably by either dry roasting or cooking them in oil, to mellow the sharp flavor of the raw seeds. It makes a good addition to meat, vegetable, and lentil dishes as well as curries. Extracts and tinctures of the spice are available as well for therapeutic use.

# Saffron (*Crocus sativus*)

Saffron, which is the stigma of the flower *Crocus sativus*, is used widely in Asia, India, and the Middle East to provide spice and a distinctive yellow color to foods. One of its main constituents, safranal, has been shown to have potent antioxidant, anti-inflammatory, antidepressant, and neuroprotective properties.[127]

## Elevates Mood

Saffron has been evaluated in multiple human studies. Five RCTs have found that saffron is effective at uplifting mood and treating moderate or major depression, functioning as effectively as prescription antidepressants; the effects are thought to be mediated by saffron's positive effect on serotonin, which is one of the brain's neurotransmitters.[128]

## Improves Alzheimer's

Other studies have showed a possible benefit in Alzheimer's disease. In one randomized, double-blind clinical trial, 30 mg per day of saffron extract was as effective as the prescription drug donepezil in treating mild to moderate Alzheimer's disease over a period of twenty-two weeks.[129] The possible mechanism for this was investigated in an animal model of Alzheimer's, in which safranal from saffron was found to protect the brain against oxidative damage.[130]

## Relieves PMS

Saffron may be beneficial in relieving symptoms of premenstrual syndrome (PMS). An RCT found that saffron was safe and effective in alleviating PMS symptoms.[131]

## Supports Fertility

Saffron is traditionally used in Ayurveda to help support healthy sexual function. At least one study provides corroborating evidence for this. In this study, 50 mg of saffron taken three times a week for three months was found to have significantly positive effect on both sperm morphology and sperm motility in men with fertility problems.[132]

### Practical Tips

Saffron has an excellent safety profile. It is usually sold in small plastic containers containing yellow-orange strands. Always soak the strands in warm water for at least five minutes before cooking to begin to release the volatile oils. Do not soak saffron in oil because that actually prevents the volatile oils from being released. For recipes using saffron, please refer to Appendix B.

## Practical Tips for Using Spices

I conclude this chapter with a few general principles about spices. Whenever a whole seed is available rather than a ground spice, I recommend purchasing the whole seed. This is because the volatile oils from spices dissipate fairly quickly once ground. More of the essential oils and nutrients, and therefore more of the therapeutic value, are retained in whole seeds rather than ground powder. Moreover, whole-seed spices have a longer half-life, generally lasting at least one year. If you do purchase ground powders, I suggest getting them in small quantities so that you go through them quickly. When you purchase whole seeds, you can grind them pretty easily using a spice grinder, a coffee grinder, or a mortar and pestle.

When cooking with spices, it's often beneficial to dry roast them in a pan to activate and release their volatile essential oils and ingredients. To do this, heat a small amount of oil such as coconut oil or olive oil in a pan. When the oil is hot, add the spices and lower the heat to medium. Stir frequently so that the spices do not get burned, and continue heating them for about a minute or two until they release their distinctive aromas.

One of the universal features of an Indian home is the (sometimes not so) faint smell of spices. The same aromatic compounds that have powerful health benefits also can make your clothes "fragrant." My job when I was young was to close all the bedroom and closet doors whenever my mom started cooking. In fact, that is still my job today when my wife starts to work her magic in the kitchen (I'm training my daughter to do this so I'll be off the hook soon)—just a practical tip to make sure your friends and coworkers do not inadvertently find out about your new love of spices through your aromatic clothing.

# PART TWO

## Exercise, Sleep, and the Mind-Body-Spirit Balance

# CHAPTER 8

# YOUR DAILY ROUTINE—AYURVEDIC TIPS AND INTERMITTENT FASTING

In this chapter, I discuss a *dinacharya,* or daily routine, based on the principles of Ayurvedic medicine. Dinacharya is important to help balance your body, regulate your natural circadian rhythm, and maintain healthy digestion. It is a ritual that provides a sense of grounding and everyday routine that can be very balancing for both body and mind. In our modern society, the power of ritual is often not utilized, and this is a simple way that you can start to incorporate basic rituals into your daily life.

The dinacharya is individualized according to your specific body type, which was determined in Chapter 2. The basic routine is listed here in sequence and explained in more detail below. Common elements for all body types include the following:

- Wake up as early as you comfortably can, preferably without an alarm clock. You should feel well rested when you arise, so go to bed earlier if you require more sleep.
- Have a tall glass of hot water with a little bit of lemon or lime juice first thing in the morning after you wake up. This is a simple beverage that strengthens your digestive fire and helps promote healthy elimination. It's best to have this drink first thing when you wake up.
- Practice oil-pulling, a technique that supports oral hygiene and detoxification.
- This should be followed by brushing your teeth and scraping your tongue, preferably with a tongue scraper, which is a U-shaped wooden or metal tool. The main benefit of tongue scraping in Ayurveda is not hygiene or cleanliness but rather stimulation of your digestive organs. The tongue is considered a microcosm of your entire body, and scraping the tongue from back to front stimulates and awakens all your organs, especially your digestive organs.
- Next, perform nasal irrigation with a neti pot and incorporate nasya; these are traditional methods to purify and revitalize the breathing

passages, reduce allergies, and decrease your chances of contracting upper respiratory infections.

- Some type of reflective or contemplative practice, even for just a few minutes, is encouraged. This could include setting some goals for the day, journaling, visualization, or a mind-body practice such as yoga, meditation, or deep breathing. This helps set the tone for the day and puts your mind in a good space as you start your morning.
- At least once a week when you have additional time (perhaps on a weekend), perform a simple Ayurvedic self-massage known as abhyanga.
- Have a shower or bath to conclude your routine.

## Oil-pulling

Oil-pulling is an ancient Ayurvedic therapy that involves holding oil in the mouth for about ten minutes and then discarding it. In Ayurveda, oil-pulling has been used to strengthen the teeth, gums, and jaws and to prevent tooth decay, gum disease, and bad breath. It is believed that oil-pulling removes toxins from the body and stimulates Agni, or digestive fire.

The practice is usually done with either sesame or coconut oil. Basically one takes about a teaspoon of oil into the mouth and swishes and "pulls" the oil around through one's teeth. After about ten minutes the oil is believed to have drawn up toxins and waste metabolites from the body and should be disposed of. Do not swallow the oil. After spitting, rinse the mouth well with water. The process should be done on an empty stomach. I would recommend starting with about five minutes of practice and slowly increasing to ten minutes.

## The Neti Pot and Nasya

The neti pot is a small pot that is designed to help cleanse your nasal passages. Fill the pot with warm water and a small amount of sea salt or Himalayan salt, about an eighth of a teaspoon. I suggest adding six to eight drops of an herbal oil known as nasya oil. This helps counteract the drying effects of the salt and provide additional calming and rejuvenating effects on the mind, in addition to other benefits.

Ayurveda considers nasya, or nasal application of oil, to be a therapy in its own right. It is often recommended for conditions such as allergies, chronic rhinitis, sinusitis, dizziness, brain fog, anxiety, and depression.[1]

The practice I have described here combines nasya with neti practice in order to save time. Nasya oil can be purchased online from companies such as Banyan Botanicals or the Ayurvedic Institute.

To use the neti pot, stand over a sink and lean your head slightly forward and to the right. Put the narrow spout of the pot into your left nostril and slowly allow the water to flow in to your nasal passageways and out your right nostril. It will take some practice. When completed, you could have the urge to blow your nose to expel additional mucus. Then tilt your head forward and to the left and insert the spout of the pot into your right nostril and repeat. Only one application in each nostril is necessary. This is especially helpful if you have allergies, sinus issues, nasal congestion, or recurrent upper respiratory infections.

## Abhyanga or Self-massage

Abhyanga is a type of Ayurvedic massage that helps to energize the mind and body, nourish the nervous system, and balance the doshas. While it is usually performed by trained Ayurvedic practitioners, self-abhyanga can be a valuable part of your daily routine. Different oils are recommended for different body types. Sesame oil is the best for vata because it has the most warming quality energetically. Coconut oil is cooling and recommended for pitta. Almond oil is stimulating and good for kapha types.

Sit or stand on a large towel spread on the floor. Use about a cup of warm oil and apply it to your entire body, starting with the head and working downward. After your head, scalp, and neck, apply oil to your shoulders, arms, chest, and abdomen. Finish by applying oil to your legs and feet, giving particular attention to your joints. Use circular movements on the torso and strokes toward the body on the arms and legs. After concluding, rest for a few minutes, and then take a shower with lukewarm water.

If you are pressed for time, applying a little oil to the top of the head and the soles of the feet is helpful and will still have significant benefit. If done at the end of the day, this practice is traditionally believed to help improve sleep.

## Meal Timing and Intermittent Fasting

Meal timing is very important in Ayurveda and is individualized according to body type. Vata types are encouraged to have regular meals and snacks when needed, while kapha types should strictly avoid snacking. Pitta types are recommended to have three meals per day at around the same time each day. There is a powerful practice known as intermittent fasting (IF) that all types can incorporate for significant benefits.

Fasting is highly regarded in Ayurvedic medicine. It is believed to stimulate the digestive fire, clear toxins, restore dosha balance, and sharpen the mind. It also helps to promote weight loss and reduce water retention as well as cleanse and tonify the vital organs and channels of the body. The Ayurvedic perspective is that the intake and digestion of food require significant amounts of energy, and when your body gets a break from this process, it can focus internally on "housecleaning" tasks such as clearing dead cells and removing toxins. From an evolutionary perspective, fasting makes sense as well. Since human beings did not have easy or continuous access to food for most of our history, we are well adapted to survive for certain periods when food is not available. During these times, our bodies can switch from burning sugar to burning fat, the most energy-rich macronutrient.

Analysis of the mealtimes and patterns of hunter-gatherers reveals that they almost never eat three meals a day plus snacks, as is typical in the United States; some commonalities that have been found include a single, large meal in the late afternoon or evening, a small breakfast that was sometimes eaten or sometimes skipped, and the notable absence of snacking.[2]

A modern, more sustainable approach that mimics this eating pattern of hunter-gatherers, while providing all the benefits of traditional fasting, is intermittent fasting (IF). This can be defined as alternating between periods of eating and periods of fasting (which might entail reduced food consumption or avoiding food completely). There are several different ways to accomplish this, as discussed below.

Intermittent fasting has been shown to help the body burn fat, increase growth hormone levels, lower triglycerides, and normalize metabolic hormones such as insulin, leptin, and ghrelin—and it does not have to be done every day to be effective. Conventional wisdom such as eating and snacking throughout the day and never skipping breakfast is outdated and inaccurate. By the way, the old advice about eating breakfast in order to help with weight loss was never proven clinically—in fact, randomized controlled trials have shown that eating breakfast has no benefit for weight loss when compared to skipping breakfast.[3]

Let us review the different types of IF and discuss which approach might be best for you depending on your Ayurvedic constitution.

## 16:8 Intermittent Fasting

One simple approach is to skip breakfast and consume all your food during an eight-hour window, usually between 12 p.m. and 8 p.m. This approach, called Leangains, was pioneered by Martin Berkhan.[4] Basically, all your calories are to be consumed in an eight-hour window later in the day, and you are to fast for the other sixteen hours. To start out, finish your dinner no later than 8 p.m. The following morning, skip breakfast—you are allowed to have black coffee or green tea—and have your first meal of the day at noon or later. If you feel dizzy or hungry, try to drink more fluids or do some light exercise. If that doesn't help, you could have a spoonful of raw extra-virgin coconut oil, which will not adversely affect the fasting phase.

To begin, try this on two nonconsecutive days of the week. As you become more comfortable, you can gradually increase the frequency of the practice. With this and all other types of IF, there is no restriction on exercise. You can continue to follow your regular exercise routine, and fasting will not have any detrimental effect on your fitness or strength gains; in fact, exercise while fasting can accelerate weight loss. 16:8 IF could potentially work well for all Ayurvedic body types.

## The 5:2 Diet or "Fast Diet"

Another approach to IF, which is popular in the UK, is described in *The FastDiet* by physician Michael Moseley.[5] This approach involves eating your typical diet for five days every week and then eating a quarter of your regular calories—500 calories for women and 600 for men—on the other two days. Case reports suggest that this is an effective way to burn fat, lose weight, and improve metabolic parameters like blood sugar and cholesterol.

One advantage of this approach is that you are still eating food on your two fasting days, just less than normal. Also, you can maintain a relatively normal diet on the other five days of the week, although it is ideal to follow Paleovedic guidelines, such as avoiding refined sugar and processed foods. This IF approach would work well for vata types, because it does not espouse complete abstinence from food and still provides some nutrition on fasting days.

## Alternate Day Fasting

If you want a more rigorous routine, or have not lost enough weight with other types of IF, you can try alternate-day fasting (ADF). This is also called the UpDayDownDay Diet, and was created by physician James Johnson.[6] In this approach, you alternate regular days with fasting days, so if you are eating your regular diet on Monday, then Tuesday would be a low-calorie day, Wednesday would be a regular day, and so forth. Therefore, you would have around three to four low-calorie days each week.

During the low-calorie days, you initially consume 500 calories for the first two weeks; after this induction phase, you can gradually increase the number of calories consumed on low-calorie days. Research on this approach shows that it is a powerful way to lose weight and improve your metabolic parameters, especially if you are starting out with more weight to lose.

## The Warrior Diet

The Warrior Diet is an advanced approach that basically involves eating one large meal every day; technically, you are allowed to have small portions of snacks during the day, so it's not strictly IF.[7] However, your main meal should be at the end of the day, and there is no restriction on quantity or type of food consumed.

This regimen is more difficult to adhere to because it allows just one meal per day, but those who are willing to follow it can derive significant benefits. This would work especially well for kapha types but would not be recommended for vata types because of the length of the gap between meals.

## Eat Stop Eat Diet

Another IF approach incorporates a complete twenty-four-hour fast, either once or twice per week. This program, called Eat Stop Eat, was developed by Brad Pilon and is well-researched and supported by a number of scientific studies.[8] Basically, it entails eating your regular diet during the other days of the week and performing a twenty-four-hour fast without food either once or twice per week. While this approach will get results, it is quite rigorous because it requires a twenty-four-hour fast, so I would not recommend it for vata body types.

As you can see, there are many different ways to practice intermittent fasting. Try out at least one or two methods to find out what works best.

## Intermittent Fasting—Benefits beyond Weight Loss

The benefits of intermittent fasting extend far beyond metabolic improvements like losing weight, improving insulin sensitivity, and lowering blood sugar, cholesterol, and triglycerides.[9] IF has significant effects on the brain through its effect on a protein known as brain-derived neurotrophic factor (BDNF). Within a few weeks, intermittent fasting raises brain levels of BDNF, which elevates mood and protects the brain against age-related mental decline and dementia.

Fasting also triggers your body to replace damaged cells and generate new red blood cells and white blood cells. Plus, it strengthens your immune system and may lower your risk of a number of different cancers. IF also leads to beneficial changes in hormones such as growth hormone. Thus, modern science has confirmed some of the traditional Ayurvedic beliefs about fasting.

Incorporating intermittent fasting and a few health-promoting Ayurvedic practices into your daily routine can offer a wide range of physical and mental benefits. Even if you are not able to incorporate all the suggestions in this chapter, adding just one or two beneficial practices to your morning ritual can be remarkably helpful.

# CHAPTER 9

# THE FIVE SECRETS OF OPTIMAL EXERCISE

For most of human history, our very survival depended on our ability to be physically active throughout the day. Daylight hours would have been spent hunting, gathering, walking, and performing manual labor. There were no couches or cars. There was no "working out"—it was just life. In today's world, this integration of exercise into our daily lives has vanished, thus making it even more important to optimize your exercise.

While government guidelines state that adults should get at least two and a half hours (150 minutes) each week of moderate-intensity aerobic physical activity, 80 percent of Americans do not meet these recommendations—and in fact 25 percent don't get any exercise at all.

This is a shame because exercise is powerful medicine. Research has demonstrated that exercise can literally change the structure of your brain by increasing the size of your hippocampus, which is important for stress management, memory, learning, and mood. Exercise can also help lower blood sugar and fasting insulin levels, promote weight loss, reduce blood pressure, raise levels of beneficial HDL cholesterol, boost your immune system, strengthen your bones, improve sleep, and increase your energy. Physical activity prevents oxidative damage and inflammation—the primary mechanisms underlying most chronic diseases like heart disease, diabetes, and cancer. Those who are sedentary have a higher risk for virtually all modern diseases. In this chapter, I reveal five secrets to optimal physical activity and exercise.

## Secret #1—Traditional Cardio Does Not Help You Lose Weight

Don't get me wrong. If you are sedentary, traditional cardio can be hugely beneficial and will improve your blood pressure, blood sugar, and lipid profile; however, studies show that the benefits of traditional cardiovascular exercise for weight loss are modest at best. Traditional cardio is any workout where you are moving steadily at a slow or moderate pace the entire time.

A high-quality review of forty-three studies on exercise concluded that the additional weight loss from traditional cardio averaged a grand total of about two pounds; they did note that higher intensity exercise was associated with more weight loss.[1]

Another reason traditional cardio is less effective for weight loss is that people may tend to consume more food after workouts due to increased appetite. So what do I recommend instead of traditional cardio workouts? Exercising the way your Paleolithic ancestors did—learning to move this way can lead to dramatic improvements in your health and vitality.

## Secret #2—Move Like Your Ancestors

High-intensity interval training (HIIT) is an approach that mimics the physical activity pattern of hunter-gatherers. Research has shown that HIIT leads to equal or superior gains in cardiovascular health and fitness when compared to traditional exercise but takes only a fraction of the time.

How did hunter-gatherers move? They didn't have access to gyms. Yet (as we saw in Chapter 1) they were extremely fit and almost entirely free of most modern chronic diseases. They performed low-intensity movements like walking, gathering foods, or manual labor daily. From time to time, the exigencies of life would require a burst of intense activity—such as going on a hunt, running from a predator, or fighting for survival.

In contrast to traditional cardio, HIIT involves performing movements at very high intensity for short periods of time—usually between thirty seconds and two minutes. Studies have been done comparing HIIT to low-intensity, steady-state exercise, and HIIT has been shown to be superior in nearly every meaningful marker. In one study, one group was assigned to traditional cardio workouts, while the other was assigned to HIIT.[2] After fifteen weeks, the researchers found that both exercise groups demonstrated a significant improvement in cardiovascular fitness. However, only the HIIT group had a significant reduction in body weight, fat mass, abdominal fat, and fasting plasma insulin levels. Leptin levels were also significantly lower in the HIIT group. Other studies have shown that high-intensity training creates uniquely favorable metabolic and structural changes in muscle.

## HIIT Burns Calories Even after You Work Out

High-intensity interval training also helps you burn calories for up to forty-eight hours after your workout is over by eliciting a powerful physiological effect known as EPOC or excess post-exercise oxygen consumption. EPOC describes your body's capacity to utilize oxygen and burn calories following a high-intensity activity. HIIT produces greater EPOC responses than traditional cardio. During the forty-eight hours after your workout, your body continues to utilize oxygen at a higher rate and burn calories by metabolizing and breaking down fat. EPOC is influenced by the intensity and not the duration of exercise, so that's why a shorter duration high-intensity workout can still have this powerful effect.

## Increase Resistance to Reduce Injuries

One way to reduce the likelihood of injury from HIIT is to use an exercise machine that allows you to control the resistance. The reason this matters is that for the moments of peak activity, if you are performing an activity that requires little resistance, you will be moving your body very quickly, as in sprints. The only concern with this is that unless you are very careful, there is more stress on your joints and a potentially higher risk of injury.

In contrast, if you use a machine such as a stationary bike or elliptical machine where you can increase the resistance, then you can still challenge your body during the high-intensity phase by maximizing the resistance but not having to move at an extremely rapid pace. Let me illustrate with an example of a HIIT workout:

- Warm up for three minutes on a cardio machine such as an elliptical machine.
- Now start your first interval of the high-intensity phase: Increase the resistance as high as tolerable such that it takes you all the effort you can muster to move for thirty seconds. You should feel like you couldn't possibly go on any longer. If you can continue moving for more than thirty seconds, it means that you need to increase the resistance.
- Lower the resistance, and move at a slow to moderate pace for ninety seconds.

- Repeat the high-intensity exercise and recovery four to five more times as tolerated. This will take you a total of about ten minutes.
- Cool down for three minutes with movement at lower resistance, and finish with stretching.

You should perform HIIT only once per week to reduce the likelihood of injury. On other days, you can perform weight training and regular low-intensity activity and movement.

## Secret #3—Be Eccentric in Your Workouts

By this I don't mean trying bizarre maneuvers but rather utilizing a very specific type of movement in strength training. I should begin by saying that strength training is absolutely essential for everyone because it promotes fat loss and builds muscle mass in addition to triggering beneficial changes in hormones such as testosterone and growth hormone. Just like HIIT, strength training also has significant EPOC and keeps your metabolism elevated post-workout. It is especially beneficial for women because it increases bone density and reduces the risk of osteoporosis and fractures. Because muscle has a higher metabolic rate than other tissues, boosting your muscle mass actually increases the number of calories you burn at rest. Government guidelines suggest that you incorporate strength training at least twice a week. You don't need to belong to a gym; you can easily do resistance training at home or outdoors.

Let me explain what I mean by an eccentric workout. In exercise physiology, there are two types of muscle movements—concentric, where the muscle is shortening during contraction, and eccentric, where the muscle is actively lengthening during contraction. Let's take the example of a bicep curl. When you are lifting the dumbbell up, the biceps muscle is shortening, and that is the concentric component. When you are lowering the dumbbell in the eccentric phase, the biceps muscle is lengthening but still contracting.

Often people emphasize the concentric phase but move very quickly through the eccentric phase, without thinking much of it. But what's more important, concentric or eccentric? The military (which does extensive research on physical fitness) can provide guidance here—the *U.S. Army Fitness Training Handbook* explains that because muscle can control more weight during the eccentric phase of contraction, eccentric training can produce greater strength gains by engaging muscle fibers more powerfully.[3]

A research review and meta-analysis of twenty trials determined that eccentric training is superior to concentric training at promoting increases in muscle strength.[4] One study showed that moving slowly during the eccentric phase (when combined with concentric exercise) can double the rates of muscle gain achieved by focusing on the concentric phase alone.[5] The take-home message is that the eccentric phase of resistance training should be emphasized and accentuated.

The way to maximize the impact of strength training is to control your movements during the entire range of motion, slowly performing both the concentric and eccentric phases. Focus on making the eccentric phase of your weight training (e.g., the downward phase of the biceps curl) last as long as possible, perhaps eight to ten seconds per repetition; this will ensure that you are maximizing the impact of the eccentric movement.

There are also specific types of weight training regimens that can be particularly beneficial, such as the eccentric weight training program of Jonathan Bailor[6] or high-intensity strength training advocated by fitness expert Doug McGuff, MD.[7] Always consult your physician before starting any exercise regimen; it may be helpful to work with a personal trainer for advanced techniques.

## Secret #4—Avoid Prolonged Sitting

Some conventional medical advice that's no longer true is the belief that going to the gym regularly is sufficient and adequate in terms of physical activity. Studies show that if you sit for long periods of time, you have an increased risk of death—even if you are exercising regularly. A large study of 220,000 adults found that sitting for eleven hours a day was associated with a 40 percent greater risk of death over just three years than sitting for less than four hours per day, regardless of whether the participants did regular exercise.[8] Reducing sitting time can significantly decrease your risk of dying from any cause, independently of your exercise routine.

Therefore, being physically active throughout the day and minimizing sitting is as important as formal exercise. Find ways to reduce sitting and inject activity into your daily routine. This could involve riding your bike as part of your commute to work, taking the stairs instead of the elevator, parking farther away from your office, and walking when you have the option rather than driving. Try to stand when you are on the bus or subway and any time you have the opportunity.

If you do have a desk job, take frequent breaks to stand up from sitting. A NASA scientist concluded that standing up from a sitting position thirty-five times per day can effectively maintain physical conditioning.[9] So standing up from a sitting position four to five times per hour can be beneficial if you are at a job that primarily requires sitting—set up a timer to remind yourself. An even better option would be to switch to a standing desk.

## Secret #5—Do Weights before Cardio

Although there is limited research on the optimal sequence of weights and cardio training, it is preferable to do your weight training before cardio. In this case, by cardio I mean HIIT or other cardiovascular workouts incorporating interval training. Again we can return to the military for guidance, as military sources recommend doing weight training first.[10] This is because the depletion of glycogen and energy stores during weight training can promote greater fat burning during subsequent cardio, and doing cardio first may reduce the efficacy of weight training by prematurely fatiguing the muscles.

Lactic acid is a by-product of oxygen depletion that is produced during anaerobic exercise such as resistance training. Performing the cardio afterward will also help to clear lactic acid, thereby reducing muscle soreness. (Stretching is another way to eliminate lactic acid.)

## Customize Your Exercise According to Ayurveda

Ayurveda has a few additional insights to offer regarding exercise. Walking is highly regarded as an excellent option for all types and is especially recommended after meals to aid digestion. Yoga is also universally recommended for innumerable physical and mental benefits. Too much exercise or exercise that's inappropriate for your constitution can be harmful.

You can individualize your exercise regimen by considering the characteristics of your Ayurvedic body type (covered in Chapter 6). Vata types are the most prone to injury and overexertion and should be careful when performing high-intensity training. Indeed, interval training with modest exertion in the intense phases—what I call moderate-intensity interval training—will be physically challenging enough for vatas and still have considerable health benefits. They are vulnerable to joint injuries and should be cautious when engaging in high-impact sports. More gentle practices such as yoga, Pilates, or tai chi are grounding and calming for vata types and should constitute the foundation of their exercise routine.

Pitta types in general love sports but should resist the tendency to become overly competitive; they may do better with team sports rather than individual sports. Water-based exercise and winter sports are considered especially beneficial for pitta. Because pitta types sweat a great deal, they should be especially careful with hydration during exercise. More restorative exercise would be a good complement to the high-intensity activities that they enjoy.

Kapha types usually dislike exercise or prefer low-impact workouts. However, vigorous exercise is essential to help stimulate and invigorate those with a kapha constitution. They are less prone to injury than other body types. High-intensity interval training and high-intensity strength training or other dynamic resistance training is especially beneficial. Having an external goal like training for a marathon can be especially motivating. Low-impact or restorative exercise is not necessary or recommended for kapha types.

For all types, the important thing is to have fun and find a type of exercise that you really enjoy. Remember that the best kind of exercise is *the kind that you will do.* Pairing up with a workout buddy or making it a family affair can provide encouragement. Increasing your activity level, both by being physically active throughout the day (i.e., sitting less!) and by participating in weight training and interval training, can lead to dramatic improvements in your health and well-being.

# CHAPTER 10
# IMPROVE YOUR SLEEP

We have a problem with widespread sleep deficiency in the United States, and most of us feel like we are not getting enough sleep. The CDC goes so far as to call insufficient sleep "a public health epidemic," not only because of accidents and injuries that result from sleep deprivation but because people who don't get enough sleep are more likely to suffer from diseases like diabetes, hypertension, obesity, depression, and cancer.[1] A line I often hear from my patients is, "I don't get enough sleep but who does? It's not a big deal." However, getting adequate sleep is absolutely fundamental to good health, and it is not possible to be healthy if you are sleep-deprived, even if your diet and physical activity are perfect.

Sleep is given short shrift because many people do not realize the proven benefits of adequate sleep:

- an increase in metabolism
- maintenance of healthy weight
- favorable changes in multiple hormones
- an improved ability to fight off infections
- sharper focus and brain function
- an enhanced ability to cope with stress
- reduced risk of multiple chronic illnesses

## The Importance of Circadian Rhythms

The human body has intrinsic rhythms just like the natural world. Circadian rhythms are your body's natural cycles that correspond to the regular patterns of daytime and night. The maintenance of normal circadian rhythms is essential for good health. When these rhythms are disrupted, health problems occur. For example, night shift workers have an increased risk over time of developing various medical problems, including heart disease, metabolic syndrome, diabetes, and certain types of cancer.[2] Factors that affect circadian rhythms include diet, sleep, sunlight exposure, and physical activity.

The primary hormone that mediates your circadian rhythms is melatonin, which is secreted by the pineal gland in the brain. This hormone has many benefits, including supporting the immune system, boosting growth hormone levels, regulating sleep, and preventing cancer. Dysregulation of melatonin is thought to be the reason night-shift workers have higher rates of cancer.

## Optimize Your Melatonin Levels

Melatonin is very important for health, immune function, and sleep quality. Hence it is critical to ensure that your melatonin levels are optimal. Unfortunately, research has shown that even exposure to ordinary room light before bedtime or during the night suppresses melatonin significantly.[3] This was not a problem for our ancestors who were not exposed to artificial light after sunset, slept in complete darkness, and synchronized their sleep-wake cycles with the rhythms of day and night.

There are steps you can take to emulate these healthy ancestral patterns. Try to keep your room as dark as possible at night, and avoid excessive exposure to lights before bedtime. The blue light from computer, TV, and cell phone screens also significantly suppresses melatonin production. Such blue light can be filtered out by wearing amber eyeglasses, which have become popular in the Paleo community; if you have to use electronics after dark, or even if you don't but you're having sleep issues, these are a good option. There are also computer programs available (such as f.lux) that can automatically dim electronic displays after dark.

## Using Diet to Regulate Circadian Rhythm

Research suggests that not just the brain but in fact every organ has its own circadian rhythm. This is consistent with Ayurveda, which states that different doshas and organs are active at different times of the day. Interestingly, fat cells have their own circadian clock, and therefore the timing of meals has important consequences on metabolic function and weight loss. For example, eating food late at night can have a disruptive effect on your circadian rhythms that can contribute to weight gain—so cut down on late-night snacks.

A study found that people who ate their main meal earlier in the day lost 25 percent more weight than people who ate their main meal later in the day (after 3 p.m.), despite consuming an identical number of calories and having similar energy expenditure.[4] This is consistent with Ayurvedic recommendations to have your main meal of the day at lunchtime, ideally before 2 p.m., and have a light dinner.

## Metabolic Hormones—Leptin and Ghrelin

The hormones leptin and ghrelin are also strongly affected by sleep. These hormones drive hunger and appetite. Leptin is produced by your fat cells and acts to increase metabolism, decrease appetite, and reduce fat deposition. Leptin also has a circadian rhythm, and levels normally peak in the middle of the night; leptin is increased by carbohydrate consumption, and therefore consuming adequate complex carbohydrates with dinner can help reinforce the natural circadian rhythm of leptin and may support healthy serotonin levels as well.[5]

Ghrelin, commonly known as "the hunger hormone," is produced by the stomach when it is empty and signals your brain to trigger the sensation of hunger. Higher levels of ghrelin trigger increased caloric intake. One study found that even a single night of sleep deprivation was able to significantly increase plasma levels of ghrelin and lead to a corresponding increase in appetite.[6] Thus, changes in metabolic hormones that result from inadequate sleep slow your metabolism and increase your appetite—thereby leading to weight gain.

Conversely, it is extremely difficult to lose weight if you are not getting adequate sleep. Studies show that lack of sufficient sleep undermines the efficacy of diet and lifestyle changes in leading to weight loss, revealing just how critical sleep is for weight regulation.[7]

## Get Some Sun during the Day

Research shows that some exposure to sunlight during the day, even through an open window, can improve your sleep by helping your body to better regulate its circadian rhythms and biological cycles.[8] If you are able to take a walk or do some exercise outdoors during the daytime, perhaps on your lunch break, that is ideal. If not, going outside to do an errand or even poking your head out a window for a bit can be helpful, as the effects of sunlight on helping regulate your circadian rhythm are very important.

It may be the ultraviolet component of sunlight that is particularly important for supporting healthy circadian rhythm. Sunlight needs to strike the retina, located in the back of your eyes, in order to signal your brain to synchronize circadian rhythm. This can be blocked by glasses or contact lenses; if possible, remove your glasses for at least part of the time that you are outside during the day to allow light to enter your eyes (but don't stare at the sun directly!). Sunlight must also strike bare skin to enable production of vitamin D, so light shining through a window is inadequate for vitamin D synthesis.

## Exercise

Exercise can definitely be helpful in improving your sleep quality. The important thing is to finish exercising at least three hours before bedtime, especially if you are performing high-intensity training. Intense exercise can raise cortisol levels, which can keep you awake if inappropriately elevated at night. Cortisol levels have a circadian rhythm and are supposed to be at their lowest during the night. If your sleep is not restful, try working out earlier in the day.

## Sleep Hygiene

There are certain recommendations for improving sleep that are known as "sleep hygiene" in medicine. These include going to bed and waking up at around the same time every day, developing a relaxing bedtime routine without electronics, and making the room slightly cool and as dark as possible when you turn in. Reserving the bedroom for sleep and sex helps your mind to associate being in bed with sleeping; therefore, it is better not to read, watch TV, or use a computer in bed.

Eating a light dinner and avoiding nighttime snacks is beneficial for multiple reasons. Reducing your intake of stimulants such as caffeine and incorporating stress reduction or relaxation techniques are useful strategies. While alcohol may help you to fall asleep, it causes a paradoxical arousal later at night and reduces the depth of sleep. It's better to avoid napping during the day unless you need to catch up on sleep or can take a short "power nap" earlier in the day that energizes you and does not disrupt your nighttime sleep.

## How Much Sleep Do I Need?

Ayurveda believes that there are significant differences in sleep requirements. Vata types need the most sleep, at least eight to nine hours. Pitta and kapha types can often do well with less sleep, in most cases seven hours and sometimes even less. The main criteria are that you should wake up feeling rested and be able to wake up naturally, without too much struggle.

## How Can I Sleep Better?

Let us review some natural strategies that can help you to sleep more soundly. The first is physical activity. It is clear that regular exercise enables people to fall asleep more quickly and to sleep more deeply. As we discussed earlier, sunlight exposure during the day (without glasses or contacts) can actually help you sleep better at night by supporting your body's circadian rhythms. Finally, reducing your exposure to artificial light at night, turning off all electronics at least two hours before bedtime, and keeping your bedroom as dark as possible will help to prevent suppression of your normal nighttime melatonin secretion.

Here are a few other techniques that can improve your sleep quality.

## Yoga

You might be surprised to see yoga discussed here and not in the chapter on physical activity. Of course, yoga is beneficial for improving flexibility, balance, and strength, and research studies have proven its effectiveness in conditions such as low back pain, arthritis, and carpal tunnel syndrome.[9] However, the benefits of authentic yoga extend beyond the physical to include mental, emotional, and spiritual effects. It can also significantly improve sleep, as many of my patients have attested. Research has confirmed this.

One randomized study in an elderly population found that yoga was able to reduce the time it took to fall asleep, increase the number of hours slept significantly, and improve the likelihood of feeling rested in the morning.[10] In a smaller study, in patients with cancer, yoga was effective at favorably affecting sleep patterns.[11] Yoga was shown to raise nighttime blood levels of melatonin in a study with healthy individuals, suggesting a possible mechanism for its enhancement of sleep.[12]

A randomized controlled study in deployed military personnel found that just three weeks of yoga was effective in reducing anxiety and significantly improving sleep; the authors found these improvements in sleep striking, given that the soldiers were experiencing "ongoing environmental disruptions to sleep from gunfire and helicopter sounds."[13] If yoga can help people sleep better under such extreme conditions, it is likely to be beneficial in routine civilian life.

Yoga is effective at inducing relaxation and activating the parasympathetic nervous system, which has physiological benefits such as reducing anxiety and lowering blood pressure, heart rate, and levels of the stress hormone cortisol. Another study in patients with depression showed that yoga was able to raise levels of the neurotransmitter serotonin and alter levels of the neurotransmitter enzyme monoamine oxidase (which is often targeted by antidepressants).[14] Therefore, yoga is an excellent option for improving quality and quantity of sleep in addition to having a favorable impact on mood and stress physiology.

## Progressive Muscle Relaxation

Progressive muscle relaxation (PMR) is another practice that can be helpful in improving sleep if practiced at bedtime. It is quite simple. The practice involves tensing and relaxing all your major muscle groups, one at a time, starting from your feet and working your way up to your head. For example, you would start with your right foot, tensing all the muscles in your foot as tightly as you can for five seconds and then relaxing completely. Then you would move to your left foot and do the same practice. Subsequently you can tense and relax your calves, thighs, buttocks, abdomen, chest, back, forearms, upper arms, neck, and head. The entire technique only takes a few minutes.

PMR is a technique that helps activate your parasympathetic nervous system and counteract the physiological effects of being in fight-or-flight, which we discuss more in Chapter 11.

Utilizing mind-body techniques and incorporating some of the simple suggestions in this chapter can help you improve the quality of your sleep and thus have a profoundly positive impact on your health. Optimal health is impossible without good sleep.

# CHAPTER 11

# THE MIND CONTROLS THE BODY: STRESS-REDUCTION AND SPIRITUALITY

Maintaining good mental and emotional health is crucial for overall wellness. This chapter starts by discussing the fight-or-flight reaction, which is a stress response that is adaptive in the short term but harmful in the long term. The problem is that poor diet, lack of sleep, and emotional stress can cause your body to stay in this "fight-or-flight" mode chronically, which is insidiously damaging. We then cover some mind-body stress-reduction techniques that you can begin practicing to counteract this.

## The Fight or Flight Reaction

The fight or flight reaction is the primal response of our nervous system that evolved to keep us alive in the jungle. When we were under threat, it enabled us to run from danger or fight for our lives. This is activated by the sympathetic nervous system, which is your body's equivalent of a gas pedal. It increases your blood pressure, speeds up your heart, raises blood sugar, and redirects blood away from your digestive tract and internal organs to your muscles so you can take action. In medical school, we learned that the sympathetic nervous system is associated with "the 4 F's"—fight, flight, fear, and sex.

There is no problem if the sympathetic nervous system is activated for short periods of time, which evolution designed it to do. The problem is that the stress of modern life leads to people being in this state most of the time. This leads to elevated levels of stress hormones such as cortisol that have harmful consequences over time, including raising blood sugar and blood pressure, promoting inflammation, suppressing the immune system, and shutting down digestion.

Your body in its wisdom does have a "brake" to counteract this—the parasympathetic nervous system. This enables your body to rest, recover, and regenerate itself. Activation of these pathways helps lower blood pressure, slow your heart rate, boost immune function, and restore digestion. All mind-body techniques have capacity to directly activate your parasympathetic nervous system, which leads to a plethora of health benefits.

## Meditation 101

The latest research from neuroscience has proven that we can literally change the structures of our brains through meditation and other practices, a concept known as neuroplasticity. For example, MRI studies revealed a significantly larger hippocampus, a region of the brain that is vital for stress management, memory, learning, and mood, and other positive changes in gray matter density after just eight weeks of meditation practice.[1] Moreover, research has shown that meditation can boost your immune system, reduce anxiety, and lower blood pressure. Meditation may improve your focus, attention span, and ability to work under stress. Daily meditation can turn on genes that reduce inflammation, fight cancer, and kill unhealthy cells. The power of the mind-body connection is immense, and can literally transform your body by modulating the expression of your DNA. I'd like to review a few common objections to starting meditation practice before discussing some techniques.

*I've tried meditation before, and my mind is all over the place, so it doesn't work for me.*

How unusual! I've never heard that before—there must be something wrong with you. But seriously, this is probably the most common objection I hear from patients. In reality, almost everyone has this experience when they first begin, because it is the nature of the mind to wander and jump around incessantly. In the Buddhist tradition, this is often described as "monkey mind."

If this happens to you, it's okay. Whenever you notice that your mind has wandered, simply bring it back to whatever you are focusing on, such as your breath or the rise and fall of your abdomen. It is this process of wandering and bringing the mind back that to me is the essence of meditation. There is no need to avoid this.

While there are certain types of meditation that emphasize concentration, the techniques I review here are more focused on awareness. All you have to do is be aware of what is going on. Therefore, there is no possibility of failure or "not doing it right." The effort you put into practice and the right intention are what matter; these will provide all the benefits.

*I relax by watching TV.*

There is a difference between active relaxation and passive relaxation, and it is important to have both in your life. Passive relaxation is when you are not engaged in any particular activity, perhaps just sitting quietly, watching a relaxing TV show, or sleeping. Active relaxation is when the mind is consciously engaged in quieting the physical and mental activity of the body. While it might seem like an oxymoron, active relaxation is actually much more powerful than passive relaxation and has profound health benefits far beyond those of passive relaxation. It helps to have both types in your life, but active mental relaxation using any of the techniques discussed below is indispensable.

*I don't have time.*

I recommend starting out with whatever you have time for, even if it's just five minutes once a day. The hardest part is starting and establishing a habit. Once you begin regular practice for some time, you'll start noticing the changes in your life. Then, it will be easier to maintain the daily routine. Any amount of meditation, no matter how short, will have some benefit.

*I already follow a religious tradition.*

Meditation is not a sectarian or religious technique. It can be practiced by people of all faiths and does not require any specific beliefs. If your religious tradition offers a type of meditation, by all means, practice it. There is no one technique that is better or worse than any other. All that matters is choosing an approach and sticking with it.

*What about mindfulness?*

Mindfulness can be defined as nonjudgmental moment-to-moment awareness. It is an approach that can be incorporated into meditation practice but can also be used to bring awareness to any moment in your daily life. A type of mindfulness practice called Mindfulness-Based Stress Reduction (MBSR) is taught in an eight-week program at many locations and is an excellent option for learning mind-body skills.

## Diaphragmatic Breathing

If you have never practiced meditation, I suggest starting with diaphragmatic breathing. You can do this in any position, but I suggest sitting comfortably in a chair or on the floor. Sit with your spine upright but relaxed. Place one hand on your abdomen and notice how your abdomen moves along with your breath. You want to have your abdomen rise when you breathe in and fall when you breathe out. This engages the diaphragm, the second-largest muscle in the body.

This is in fact opposite to how many people breathe. Often when you breathe in, your chest and shoulders rise up and your abdomen is drawn inward. If you look at how newborn babies breathe, they usually breathe using their diaphragms. As we have gotten older, we have forgotten how to breathe!

Diaphragmatic breathing has been shown to activate your parasympathetic nervous system and has numerous benefits, such as lowering blood pressure and reducing cortisol levels. To begin, try to practice for about five minutes and observe how you feel afterward. This is a technique that you can perform any time, while stopped at a red light in the car, while waiting in line at the grocery store, or at night before you are going to sleep (it might help you sleep better).

## Breathing Awareness Meditation

This is a simple technique that involves being aware of your breath. To begin, sit comfortably with your spine erect but relaxed. You can either close your eyes or keep a gentle gaze on a point in front of you.

Start by focusing your attention on your breath, wherever you notice it in your body. You may observe the air passing through your nostrils or the rise and fall of your abdomen. Simply observe your breathing without trying to make it any particular way. Do not try to change the way you are breathing. If you like, you could mentally say something like "breathing in" as you breathe in and "breathing out" when you breathe out.

Whenever your mind wanders (as it surely will), simply notice it and bring it back to focus on your breathing. Do not be too upset or frustrated if you are not able to keep your attention on your breathing. This does not mean you are doing it wrong. The very process of bringing your focus back to your breath, over and over, is the practice of meditation. Start with five minutes of practice and gradually increase to fifteen minutes a day, which is what I recommend for most people.

## Use an App

There are many useful apps for meditation, such as Headspace, Calm, and Insight Timer. I like the app Buddhify because it has a visually attractive interface and has recordings that you can listen to corresponding to different scenarios you might find yourself in throughout the day, like waiting in line or riding to work on the subway—opportunities for what they call "urban meditation." You can try out different apps to see what works best for you.

## Pranayama

Ayurvedic science features a vast array of different breathing exercises collectively known as pranayama. I would like to discuss one type of pranayama known as alternate-nostril breathing, which is very calming for the mind and body and helps with balancing the doshas.

Sit comfortably with your spine erect but relaxed. You can either close your eyes or keep a gentle gaze on a point in front of you. Start by using your right ring finger to cover up your left nostril. Take a deep breath in through your right nostril to a count of four. Then cover your right nostril with your thumb and hold your breath for a count of eight. Then release your left nostril and exhale to the count of four. Next, inhale through your left nostril to a count of four, hold a count of eight, and exhale through your right nostril to a count of four. You have just completed one cycle. To start, complete around five cycles, and gradually increase up to ten cycles per session. It can be a powerful practice, so if you feel dizzy at any time, just stop and take a break. For detailed instructions about this and other types of pranayama, please visit my website.

There are several other strategies that can be helpful in supporting emotional and psychological health.

## Maintain a Positive Attitude

The importance of cultivating a positive attitude was instilled in me from a young age by my father, who taught me many valuable lessons. The Indian teacher Paramahansa Yogananda, whose autobiography so impressed Steve Jobs that he arranged for it to be given to all attendees at his memorial service,[2] wrote, "Avoid a negative approach to life. Why gaze down the sewers when there is loveliness all around us? One may find some fault in even the greatest masterpieces of art, music, and literature. But isn't it better to enjoy their charm and glory? Life has a bright side and a dark side . . . Look only for the good in everything."[3]

From a utilitarian perspective, this has a surprisingly large effect on health. Research shows that a positive attitude has substantial health benefits. A review of eighty-three scientific studies showed that optimists enjoy better health than pessimists in areas such as longevity, cancer survival, and immune function, as well as outcomes related to pregnancy, physical symptoms, and pain.[4] Some strategies to increase optimism include focusing on the positive, noticing and letting go of negative self-talk, avoiding dwelling on setbacks and past hardships, thinking of things you are grateful for, appreciating others, and reframing how you define events—for example, thinking of something as a learning experience rather than a failure.

## Manage Your Emotions Well

The importance of managing your emotions well cannot be overemphasized. In my clinical experience, emotional stress is one of the most difficult issues for people to deal with—in comparison, diet and exercise are relatively easier. There many different ways to learn to manage your emotions effectively. In our society, we do not have much training or education on how to do this. Working with a psychotherapist or counselor, reading books about this topic, and journaling can help improve our skills.

Not repressing your feelings but rather accepting and experiencing them is a sensible approach. When you are faced with difficult emotions, diaphragmatic breathing, pranayama, meditation, or intense exercise (depending on the emotion) can be helpful. Once they have run their course, the emotions will change and eventually move on. Learning to handle your emotions skillfully can yield valuable rewards for overall well-being.

## Gratitude and Forgiveness

Gratitude and forgiveness are two other extremely powerful practices. Research on gratitude supports significant benefits including an increased sense of well-being, improved relationships, and a greater sense of happiness.[5] Please see the following box for some ideas about how to practice gratitude.

Forgiveness is also a valuable practice that is positively associated with mental health outcomes such as increased psychological well-being, cognitive flexibility, and happiness.[6] It can be applied to oneself, others, and possibly even life situations.

**Ideas on Practicing Gratitude**

1. Write a short email expressing your gratitude to someone in your life once a week, being specific about things you appreciate about them. Thank them for the things that they do that make your life better in some way. If you're ambitious, you could try doing this exercise daily.

2. Keep a gratitude journal. Write detailed descriptions each day of one or two things that you are grateful for. Every so often, challenge your mind to come up with a longer list, perhaps thirty or more items.

3. Before going to bed, review your day and reflect on two things you are grateful for. The key with all these methods is that you have to be as specific and detailed as possible; granular recollections are more potent than generalities. Just thinking that you are grateful for good health and your family, for example, may not be very impactful. On the other hand, if you remember a moment during your day in which your daughter smiled at you and you realized how much you loved her and how grateful you are for that connection, that is much more compelling.

## Your Sugar Pill Is Ready—Placebos and Healing

One of the most interesting aspects of mind-body research is the effect of placebos. While the definition of placebo is an inner substance that has no effect, scientific studies consistently show that placebos have a real and measurable therapeutic effect. There are many things that can contribute positively to the placebo effect, such as the white coat of a doctor or a patient's expectation about a medication.

Also, there is a difference in terms of degree of effect. Someone who believes they are getting a high-quality treatment rather than a low-quality treatment will likely have larger improvement, even if both treatments are placebos. For example, one study told patients with Parkinson's disease that they would receive either an expensive or cheap new medication; both "medications" were simply saline injections. Patients who were told they were receiving the expensive treatment exhibited greater improvement in tremor and muscle stiffness than patients who were told they were receiving the cheap medicine.[7]

In fact, some conventional treatments may work either mostly or entirely as a result of the placebo effect. For example, in patients with mild to moderate depression, the effect of antidepressant medication is comparable to a placebo (but they both work).[8]

Also, "placebo surgery" was shown to be as effective as regular surgery in some cases. To study the effects of arthroscopic surgery of the knee for osteoarthritis, researchers randomized patients to receive either traditional knee arthroscopy with debridement or a sham surgery in which the usual knee incisions were made under anesthesia and all aspects of the regular operation were simulated. At the end of one year and two years, pain reduction and improvement in physical function were identical in patients who received actual knee surgery and patients who received sham surgery.[9] The interesting thing was that about 13 percent of patients from both groups believed they had received the placebo surgery, so patients really could not tell whether they had actually received the surgery or not—but they got better either way.

The fascinating lesson here is that your body has an incredible ability to heal itself, especially when it believes that it should be healing, such as after knee surgery. The power of belief, expectation, and hope to translate into measurable physical differences is profound. I find it amazing that the mind has the capacity to affect the physical body in such a significant way. Instead of rejecting placebos as useless, we should take advantage of them. We should use every opportunity we can to help people develop the belief that they are going to get better and that they should in fact expect themselves to recover from disease and illness.

Harvard researcher Ted Kaptchuk has done some pioneering work on placebos. In one study, he demonstrated that patients with irritable bowel syndrome (IBS) improved significantly on placebos *even when they were told they were taking a placebo.*[10] In this case, patients were told they were being given inert placebo pills but were also told that placebos could potentially improve IBS symptoms "through mind-body self-healing processes"; 60 percent of placebo recipients improved, compared to only 35 percent of patients in the "no treatment" group. The power of positive expectation may be a big part of how placebos work.

Of course, placebos are not a cure for everything. However, it is a good idea for you to do whatever you can to feel good about your body and expect that it will heal itself as much as possible from afflictions. The body has phenomenal self-healing capacity. Believing that you will get better can be powerful medicine.

## Find Ways to Get Connected

As we discussed in Chapter 1, social connectedness and a strong sense of community are foundational to exceptional longevity. In modern society, we have an epidemic of social isolation and disconnectedness. Not surprisingly, we also have rampant depression and mood disorders. One of the most important things you can do for your health is to improve your social connections. For ideas on how to do this, please refer to the end of Chapter 1.

## Cultivate a Sense of Spirituality

It is important to develop a sense of spirituality. Spirituality is whatever gives you a sense of meaning, purpose, and direction in your life. It may or may not have anything to do with religion. For many of my patients, organized religion is unappealing and may have negative connotations. If you are part of a religious community that you feel connected to, that is wonderful. I encourage you to deepen your connection with your faith and develop that aspect of your life.

If you do not consider yourself a religious person, and even if you are an atheist, it is possible to cultivate a sense of spirituality. In fact, it is one of the most important things you can do for your health and is something that is commonly neglected by people in our fast-paced world. Just as with optimism, research attests to the positive effects of spirituality on a variety of health outcomes.[11]

We all need a sense of purpose in life, a reason to wake up in the morning. If you are not sure what gives you a sense of purpose and direction, it can be helpful to spend some time reflecting on this question. In fact, setting some time aside regularly to spend in introspection about the trajectory of your life can provide valuable perspective. Writing in a journal, talking with a close friend or family member, or allowing downtime for ideas to percolate are some ways to engage these questions. Finding a definitive answer is not as important as allowing time to contemplate these issues—the answers will become clearer over time.

Again, it is important to incorporate a sense of lightness and fun into this process. Often people think of spirituality as a serious and heavy topic, and it can be. But when trying to engage questions about purpose and direction in life, it is helpful to maintain a curious, playful perspective, the way a child explores something new. This makes it easier to continue engaging these questions on an ongoing basis.

## Age Is a Mental State

What I have seen in my work with patients is that age is less important when people are engaged in projects or activities that they find very meaningful. I have many patients in their seventies, officially past retirement age, who are still busy with work that they really enjoy and show no signs of slowing down. Often, they love what they're doing and do not consider it "work."

"Age isn't as important so long as you are surrounded by people you love, doing things you passionately believe in," said the entrepreneur Richard Branson.[12] I believe this is critical. The other aspect that is important is to have fun and to maintain a sense of humor about what you are doing. It is important not to take yourself too seriously and to be able to laugh at yourself occasionally. Doing things that are fun, both at work and outside of work, is essential. It is something that successful people often make time for, no matter how busy their schedule is.

Regarding the issue of age, I do not believe that has to limit you. There are many well-known stories of people who have succeeded later in life. For example, Colonel Sanders, the founder of Kentucky Fried Chicken, was in his mid-sixties when he developed his recipe for fried chicken and began trying to sell it to stores. He was rejected over and over, but he remained persistent and eventually became a tremendous success.

Age should not be used as an excuse for not feeling well. In my practice, I do not accept the excuse "I must be getting old" as an explanation for any symptom. It is quite possible for people to feel well at any age as long as the elements of health are present. Functional medicine can be helpful. For example, I have a few patients in their seventies who complained of fatigue and had subtle abnormalities in thyroid hormones that were not considered significant. When I optimized their thyroid function, they reported remarkable improvements in energy and overall vitality.

## Conclusion

In summary, practicing regular stress-reduction techniques, maintaining a positive attitude, and cultivating a sense of meaning and purpose in your life are critical for good health. There are many different ways to accomplish this. If you are not sure where to begin, simply make the commitment that this is a priority, and begin to explore these areas in ways that we have discussed in this chapter. The specific details will start to fall into place over time.

# PART THREE

## Detoxify to Reach the Next Level of Health

# CHAPTER 12
# REDUCING YOUR EXPOSURE TO TOXINS

The challenge of modern times is the ubiquity of toxins in our water, food, air, and environment. Chronic, low-level exposure is the norm for all of us. Addressing this area can have major clinical impact and is often not emphasized enough.

There are different categories of toxins, including food toxins, industrial chemicals like pesticides, and heavy metals such as lead and mercury. There are over 85,000 chemicals registered with the Environmental Protection Agency for industrial use, and most have not been studied for long-term safety. As with all potential toxins, the important issue is the cumulative dose. Many of these chemicals may become problematic after building up in the body over a number of years through a process known as bioaccumulation. Therefore, it is beneficial to try to reduce your exposure to chemicals and toxins as much as possible.

## Do Toxins Really Matter?

Do industrial chemicals have real health effects, and do we really need to worry about them? Shouldn't our bodies be able to clear chemicals without suffering any adverse consequences? Unfortunately, studies indicate that the effects of toxins are indeed real. A variety of endocrine-disrupting chemicals (EDCs) were linked to earlier menopause in one study with 30,000 women.[1] EDCs are implicated in a wide variety of health conditions, including obesity, diabetes, infertility, cancer, and neurological disease.[2] BPA used to line canned foods was shown in one randomized study to increase blood pressure.[3] Pesticides have been linked to multiple cancers, Parkinson's disease, low birth weight, birth defects, and low sperm count.[4] More studies are discussed later in this chapter.

In my practice I see many patients in whom environmental toxins have a significant detrimental effect. There is also a wide variability in how well people are able to process and clear toxins. There is a highly individual response to toxic load—for one person, a slight increase in body levels of mercury can be seriously disabling and result in many different symptoms, while a different person could be asymptomatic despite having much higher levels of mercury. There are many factors that are responsible for these differences, including genetics, nutritional status, liver function, and variability in an important set of processes known as methylation.

## Say Hello to Your Liver . . .

The liver is your main defense against toxins. In addition to helping with digestion, the liver is the primary organ responsible for filtering the blood and removing toxins. Many toxins are fat-soluble, and these toxins are stored in body fat and cell membranes, which are primarily consumed of lipids. This makes it hard for the body to eliminate such toxins. The liver must convert such fat-soluble toxins into water-soluble forms that can be excreted from the body.

It does this through a two-step process called Phase 1 and Phase 2 detoxification. Phase 1 is carried out by an enzyme known as cytochrome P450. This system processes toxins into intermediate metabolites that could be highly reactive or harmful unless they are broken down by Phase 2 pathways. Phase 2 requires combining the intermediate compounds with other molecules in a process known as conjugation, thus creating water-soluble by-products. In Phase 2, the intermediates can be conjugated with any one of the following—glucuronide, sulfate, methyl groups, amino acids, acetyl groups, or glutathione. These end-products are removed from the body either by the kidneys through urine or by the intestines via bile and stool. Interestingly, the microbiome also plays an important role in the process of detoxification.

### How Gut Bacteria Affect Detoxification and Cancer Risk

As with almost every bodily process, detoxification is affected by the microbiome. The primary way this occurs is through an enzyme known as beta-glucuronidase, which is normally present in the intestine but can be produced in high levels by certain pathogenic bacteria. Why does this matter? Remember how we talked about Phase 2 liver enzymes and that one of the pathways involves combining the intermediate compound with glucuronide? The addition of glucuronide is what allows these substances to be excreted into the stool where they can be expelled from the body. However, beta-glucuronidase is an enzyme that cleaves and removes the glucuronide, thereby allowing reabsorption of molecules that were supposed to be eliminated from the body. Environmental toxins could thus be reabsorbed.

The liver also plays a role in hormone balance, processing and excreting excess estrogen by linking it with glucuronide. Therefore, abnormal gut bacteria that increase beta-glucuronidase disrupt estrogen excretion, allowing it to be reabsorbed and contributing to excess levels of this hormone. Elevated levels of intestinal beta-glucuronidase have been linked to increased risk of hormone-dependent cancers such as breast and prostate cancer.[5] There is also a strong association between beta-glucuronidase and colon cancer.[6] It is possible through functional medicine testing to measure the level of beta-glucuronidase in the stool, which helps gauge the health of the microbiome and also assess colon cancer risk to some degree. The good news is that interventions that benefit the microbiome, including dietary modifications and probiotics, can bring down elevated levels of beta-glucuronidase and thereby reduce cancer risk and enable better clearance of toxins from the body.

As with all things in the body, there is a fine line between too little and too much beta-glucuronidase, which is present not just in the intestine but in the liver and other organs as well. The enzyme should be active enough to help break down toxic chemicals and allow absorption of certain beneficial substances without being so high that it enables reabsorption of toxins and hormones.

Phase 1 and Phase 2 have to be optimally balanced—if the reactive metabolites produced by Phase 1 are not quickly broken down, they can build up and cause cellular damage or uncomfortable symptoms such as headaches, fatigue, dizziness, stomach upset, aches and pains, or nausea. Therefore, it is crucial to support both Phase 1 and Phase 2 while doing any type of detoxification. What we commonly see in our practice is relative overactivity of the

Phase 1 pathway and underactivity of Phase 2. This can sometimes produce symptoms such as fatigue, malaise, or excessive reactivity to chemicals.

## Foods That Help You Detoxify

Grapefruit juice is a well-known modulator of Phase 1 enzymes and has phytochemicals that can reduce the activity of cytochrome P450. In fact, it is so effective that doctors recommend avoiding grapefruit juice if you are taking certain pharmaceuticals because it can affect blood levels of drugs that are metabolized by Phase 1 liver pathways.

Consuming cruciferous vegetables, such as cauliflower, broccoli, and brussels sprouts, is particularly good for both Phase 1 and Phase 2 pathways. You might recall that sulfate addition was one of the Phase 2 pathways mentioned above—support for this pathway comes from sulfur-rich foods such as garlic, eggs, onions, shallots, and leeks.

Beet greens, the leafy tops of beets, are the richest food source of betaine (also known as trimethylglycine), a powerful detoxifying compound that aids methylation and supports Phase 2 pathways. Beet greens are one of the most powerful foods to aid in detoxification. Many vitamins and minerals are key cofactors for the enzymes involved in liver detox.

Turmeric is beneficial in detoxification because it inhibits Phase 1 and stimulates Phase 2, which helps neutralize and clear the reactive intermediate compounds produced by Phase 1. Milk thistle (*Silybum marianum*) is a commonly used herb that has been shown to protect the liver in both animal and human studies through multiple mechanisms including support of both Phases 1 and 2.[7]

## Heavy Metals

Heavy metals have unfortunately become a widespread environmental problem. Mercury is present in dental fillings, fish, and seafood, and in low levels in certain water sources. Mercury is present in high amounts in certain people, and it is possible to test for this with functional medicine.

Research on mercury reveals the remarkable ways that it can damage health, with particular implications for autoimmune disease. Specifically, mercury reacts with certain proteins in the body by combining directly with body tissue. The result is a complex hybrid that is heavy metal plus body cell, an unbelievable half-human, half-metal chimera.[8] Naturally, the immune system recognizes this as a foreign invader, creating antibodies against this partially human tissue. These antibodies lead the immune system to attack this hybrid protein but can also coordinate an immune attack on our own cells. This is partly why mercury is implicated as a potential cause in the increasing epidemic of autoimmune disease.

Lead is another heavy metal that has toxic effects. Sources of lead exposure include plumbing in older houses, lead paint, canned foods, and certain types of cookware. Unfortunately, it is possible that the slow cooker you are using to cook foods in a healthy way may be a source of lead contamination. Some data suggest that certain slow cookers may leach low levels of lead into the food, especially if acid-containing foods such as vinegar, citrus, or tomato products are cooked in them. An investigation in Utah found that 20 percent of slow cookers were releasing measurable amounts of lead into foods; this is thought to be due either to the glaze that lines the vessels or something in the vessels themselves.[9] While it is possible that your slow cooker may not have this issue, I have personally stopped using my traditional slow cooker.

Safer options for cookware include glass, cast-iron, enameled cast-iron, and stainless steel. Because of potential toxicity, you want to avoid cookware that has a traditional nonstick coating such as Teflon, the brand name for a chemical known as polytetrafluoroethylene (PTFE); perfluorooctanoic acid (PFOA) is a compound used in the production of Teflon that also has possibly toxic effects. WearEver Pure Living cookware, which features a nonstick ceramic coating free of lead, cadmium, PTFE, and PFOA, is another good option.

## Food Toxins—Pesticides

Whenever possible, I recommend eating organic food to reduce pesticide exposure. The nonprofit Environmental Working Group releases an annual guide to pesticide residues and foods.[10] The guide ranks forty-eight popular fruits and vegetables based on an analysis of 32,000 samples tested by government agencies. Unfortunately, 65 percent of produce samples analyzed by the US Department of Agriculture test positive for pesticide residues.[11]

Pesticides have been linked to multiple types of cancer, Parkinson's disease, birth defects, and low sperm count, among other health problems; in 2003, the CDC determined that 93 percent of Americans tested had detectable levels of the insecticide chlorpyrifos, and 99 percent had detectable levels of a metabolite of DDT, with the average person carrying about thirteen pesticides.[12] This is concerning because the CDC tests for only a fraction of the total number of pesticides to which we are exposed but still found that a significant number of people tested had potentially harmful body levels of certain pesticides above government safety thresholds. Little research has been done on the possible synergistic effects of multiple pesticides in the body.

Children may be particularly vulnerable. The American Academy of Pediatrics issued a report asserting that children have "unique susceptibilities to [pesticide residues'] potential toxicity."[13] The pediatricians' organization cited research that linked pesticide exposures in early life to "pediatric cancers, decreased cognitive function, and behavioral problems." Studies have shown that organic produce, as you would expect, is consistently much lower in pesticide residues. Research has also shown, with few exceptions, that organic produce is higher in vitamins and minerals than conventional fruits and vegetables.

## Food Toxins—Genetically Modified Foods (GMOs)

Another aspect of toxins in foods is the controversial issue of genetically modified (GM) foods. Genetic modification basically involves inserting DNA from a different plant or animal into the DNA of a particular organism. While the original idea behind genetic modification of foods came from an attempt to address issues of world hunger, there is some evidence that suggests that these foods are not benign and may have unpredictable adverse consequences. Since these are novel new types of food that our bodies have never been exposed to, you would think that there would be extensive regulation and third-party testing. However, independent third-party testing is limited, as most of the research is funded by the companies producing the products.

French researchers reviewed the industry research on genetically modified foods and found a number of flaws in the studies and potential risks for liver and kidney toxicity from GM organisms (GMOs).[14] In lab studies, some residues present in GM foods can disrupt the endocrine system at levels hundreds of times below what is present in GM foods and can cause DNA damage and inhibition of enzyme activity.[15]

Widely grown "Bt" crops are plants that have been genetically engineered to produce the insecticidal bacteria-derived toxin bacillus thuringiensis (Bt); it was believed that Bt toxins were broken down in the GI tract and not absorbed, but studies have demonstrated the presence of Bt toxins produced by GM foods in the blood of both pregnant women and their fetuses.[16] Bt toxins are not inert to human cells and have been shown to have significant and sometimes toxic effects on human cells, such as triggering cell death.[17] But residues cannot be washed off because they are produced by the plants themselves within their own cells. GM corn is pervasive in the US food supply as animal feed, high fructose corn syrup, and a key ingredient in many processed foods.

Another concern is the effect of GMOs on the gut microbiome. Studies have shown that it is possible for bacteria typically found in the human gut to take on genes from GM foods through a process known as gene transfer.[18] Therefore, genetically modified foods have the potential to change the genetic makeup of the bacteria that comprise your microbiome, which affect almost every process in your body—the long-term effects of such genetic changes have never been studied and are unknown.

## Glyphosate and GMOs

Glyphosate is the world's most commonly used pesticide, owned and produced by Monsanto under the name Roundup. Global glyphosate demand is estimated at 770,000 tons (about 1.5 *billion* pounds) for 2016.[19] Genetically engineering glyphosate-resistant genes into common food crops enables glyphosate to be used liberally and at higher doses, likely leading to higher glyphosate residues on the crops; glyphosate residues in wheat and other crops may be increasing as a result of agricultural practices such as crop desiccation.[20] Also, weeds are becoming resistant to glyphosate, requiring application of larger quantities of the pesticide.

What are the health effects of glyphosate? Glyphosate is known to cause DNA damage and potentially induce cell death in human cells; it may be a contributing factor to Parkinson's disease, Alzheimer's disease, depression, infertility, and gastrointestinal disorders; and it is known to disrupt the endocrine system as well, potentially affecting hormone levels.[21] According to an MIT researcher, glyphosate inhibits the cytochrome P450 liver enzymes, which are critical for breaking down environmental toxins and excess hormones, and adversely affects the amino acid synthesis of our gut bacteria.[22] It is also known to damage the microbiome by causing a decline in beneficial bacteria and predisposing to overgrowth of pathogenic bacteria.[23]

There is a potential link between glyphosate and certain cancers. A Swedish study found that patients with non-Hodgkin's lymphoma were three times more likely to report previous exposure to glyphosate.[24] There was an association between glyphosate exposure and multiple myeloma in US pesticide applicators.[25] Glyphosate has been labeled a "probable carcinogen" by experts from the World Health Organization.[26] To be fair, there are some reviews that claim that glyphosate is safe and has no long-term human toxicity whatsoever.[27]

So what is the verdict? The jury is still out, as there are a number of question marks in the scientific literature as well as multiple conflicting studies and broader concerns about industry bias in the research. My approach with chemicals is to try to reduce our exposure to them, because our bodies have to deal with such a large number of them every day in our environment—so it is preferable to minimize GMO intake. Unfortunately, glyphosate residues cannot be washed off of food crops, so it is best to avoid foods that normally contain it, especially conventionally grown soy, corn, and wheat.

There is no food labeling requirement that foods containing GMOs have to be labeled as such. Legislation to require such labeling, as was previously proposed in California, has frequently been defeated with extensive lobbying from the food industry; recent exceptions are Connecticut, Maine, and Vermont, which are trying to mandate a degree of labeling. The most well-established regulation pertaining to GMOs is organic certification—foods that are certified USDA organic are not allowed to have GMO ingredients. The nonprofit Non-GMO Project enables foods to be labeled with a "Non-GMO Project Verified" seal to help consumers distinguish between GMO and non-GMO foods.

While the prevailing industry view is that lack of data proving toxicity implies that GMO foods are safe, long-term studies are needed to investigate and truly determine the safety of GMOs. It is impossible to avoid GMOs completely because of their pervasiveness in our food supply. My advice is to try to limit your exposure to them when possible, because the fewer potentially toxic chemicals you are exposed to, the better.

## Toxins—Endocrine Disrupting Chemicals

Endocrine disrupting chemicals, or EDCs, are used extensively in agriculture, consumer products, cosmetics, furniture, electronics, and other industrial applications. EDCs are known to disrupt the function of the human endocrine system, which consists of the glands that produce hormones that regulate metabolism, growth and development, tissue function, sexual function, sleep, and mood, among other things. Scientists have estimated the health-care costs associated with the effects of EDCs to be a staggering $175 billion per year in Europe alone; this is one reason the European Union is considering regulation of EDCs.[28] Examples of endocrine disrupting compounds are pesticides, BPA, phthalates, and flame retardants.

## Toxins—BPA and BPA Substitutes

BPA, or bisphenol A, is a hormonally active chemical that is a known EDC; the US Centers for Disease Control and Prevention estimates that five to six billion pounds of BPA are produced worldwide each year.[29] Studies show that 93 percent of people in the United States have detectable levels of BPA in their body.[30]

You have probably seen signs for BPA-free products, which are ostensibly safer. In these products, BPS is often used as a substitute for BPA. Unfortunately, some research suggests that BPS may have toxic effects as well.[31] In animals, exposure to BPS causes irregular heartbeats, the same way that BPA does, by affecting the response of the cells to estrogen. This is not surprising because the chemical structure of BPS is similar to BPA. Further research is needed to investigate the potential toxicity of BPS and other BPA substitutes found in BPA-free products.

## Daily Detoxification

Let us review some simple, effective strategies for daily detoxification. These include incorporating specific foods and supplements and other beneficial approaches in order to reduce the buildup of toxins in our bodies. With toxins it is a simple equation:

Toxins in – Toxins out = Toxic Load

Therefore, it is beneficial to try to reduce your exposure to chemicals as much as possible (the intake side of the equation). This is complemented by regular detoxification, both regular gentle practices and periodic intensive cleansing, which comprise the "toxins out" component. We begin by discussing strategies to reduce exposure to household and environmental toxins.

## Reducing Exposure to Toxins

1. Minimize exposure to mercury.
    - Studies show that heavy metals such as mercury are prevalent in water and certain foods, especially larger fish. Mercury has harmful effects on various body systems, including the nervous system and immune system.
    - If you have mercury-containing dental amalgam fillings, consider working with a holistic dentist to have them replaced with safer composite materials. Work with a functional medicine practitioner to provide detox support during this process.
    - Choose low-mercury fish (wild salmon, mackerel, sardines, flounder), and avoid high-mercury fish (swordfish, tuna, orange roughy, marlin, shark).
    - When taking a fish oil supplement, select a product that has been third-party tested for heavy metals (e.g., Nordic Naturals, Carlson).
    - Avoid bottled water, spring water, or tap water. Drink water purified by a reverse osmosis water filtration system. Units that can be

installed under your sink are available from Costco. If you live in an apartment, portable reverse osmosis systems are available.

2. Minimize exposure to lead.
    - Ensure that your house is free of lead-based paint.
    - If you are in an older home, make sure there is no lead plumbing.
    - Avoid using a slow cooker or any pots with a glazed surface. Safer options for cookware include glass, cast-iron, enameled cast-iron, and stainless steel.
    - If you consume canned food, transfer the food after opening the can to a different (preferably glass) container before storing in the refrigerator.

3. Purchase organic fruits and vegetables whenever possible.
    - The Environmental Working Group releases a list of fruits and vegetables called "The Dirty Dozen" that have the highest pesticide residues even after cleaning and washing at home. Try to always purchase organic versions of these:
        - apples, strawberries, grapes, spinach, celery, tomatoes, green peppers, chili peppers, potatoes, cucumbers, nectarines, and green leafy vegetables like kale and collard greens
    - The same group also identified fifteen vegetables called "The Clean Fifteen" that have the lowest pesticide residues. It is acceptable to purchase conventional versions of these if you are not able to get organic for whatever reason:
        - corn, onions, pineapple, avocado, cabbage, frozen peas, papaya, mangoes, asparagus, eggplant, kiwi, grapefruit, sweet potato, cantaloupe, and cauliflower

4. Green your household chemicals.
    - According to the Environmental Protection Agency, chemicals released into our homes by home care products can make indoor air five times more polluted than the air we breathe outdoors.
    - Choose household cleaners that are free of toxins. Many natural brands are available (e.g., Seventh Generation, Biokleen). You can also make your own household cleaners using ingredients like white distilled vinegar and baking soda.

- When painting, select paints with low levels of volatile organic compounds (VOCs).
- When bringing back clothes from the dry cleaner, allow them to air out in a garage or well-ventilated space before putting them in your closet. This will allow the clothes to release chemicals used during dry cleaning so they do not accumulate in your closet.

5. Update your personal grooming products and practices.
   - To evaluate your cosmetics, visit www.safecosmetics.org or www.ewg.org/skindeep.
   - Select antiperspirant that does not contain aluminum, a heavy metal that is difficult to clear from the body.
   - When choosing skin-care products, shaving creams, or cosmetics, choose natural products that do not contain parabens, phthalates, toluene, synthetic colors or fragrances, or other artificial ingredients.
   - Install a shower filter. Unfortunately it's possible to absorb significant quantities of chemicals such as chorine and chloramines through typical showers. A good quality shower filter, which you can install yourself, can prevent this. Good brands include Aquasana and Berkey.
   - Change to a fluoride-free toothpaste. Many people get adequate fluoride intake through the water supply, and excess fluoride can inhibit the thyroid and have other harmful effects. Remember the dentist Weston Price from Chapter 1? His work showed that dental health is closely tied to nutritional status, and cavities are more likely related to refined sugar intake and mineral deficiencies than a lack of fluoride.
   - Minimize nail polish, which contains phthalates, formaldehyde, and toluene.

6. Reduce exposure to flame retardants.
   - Flame retardants are ubiquitous chemicals in couches, cushions, and mattresses that are known disruptors of the endocrine system.
   - Look for organic and "green" building materials, carpeting, baby items, mattresses, and upholstery. Furniture products filled with cotton, wool, or polyester tend to be safer than chemical-treated polyurethane foam; some products also state that they are "flame-retardant free."
   - PBDEs are often found in household dust, so clean your home with a HEPA-filter vacuum and/or a wet mop often.

- Research has shown that washing your hands frequently (and especially before meals) reduces body levels of flame retardants, since we often pick up small amounts of these chemicals on our hands through contact with objects at home or at work throughout the day—and transfer them to our mouth inadvertently.[32] Another study found that children who washed their hands at least five times a day had levels of fire retardants on their hands 30 to 50 percent lower than children who washed their hands less frequently.[33] Washing your hands regularly is an easy way to reduce exposure to these chemicals.

## Practice Regular Detoxification

With the prevalence of chemicals in our environment, it is impossible to avoid exposure completely. Regular detoxification is important to help consistently reduce our body burden of these chemicals.

## Keep Your Liver Healthy

As we discussed, the liver is the most important organ in your body for detoxification. Keep your liver in good shape by following these guidelines:

1. Avoid excessive acetaminophen consumption. Acetaminophen is sold under the well-known brand name Tylenol, but is also available as a generic or store brand, and may be an ingredient in other medications such as cold medicines. Read product labels to determine acetaminophen content.

2. Drink alcohol only in moderation (e.g., no more than one to two glasses of red wine per day).

3. Talk to your doctor to see if screening blood tests to evaluate your liver function would be appropriate for you, especially if you take prescription drugs.

4. Consider being vaccinated for hepatitis A and hepatitis B.

5. Perform more intensive detoxification programs at least twice a year under the supervision of your health-care practitioner.

## Take Advantage of Sweating to Detoxify

The skin is your largest organ. The skin tends to absorb a fair amount of anything applied topically, which is why it is important to use natural skin-care products. In addition, the skin can be used for detoxification:

1. Sweating is an effective way to release toxins that are stored in the subcutaneous fat layer just underneath our skin. To do this, sweating must result from the body being gradually heated from an external source. Therefore, sweating from exercise does not accomplish as much in terms of detoxification, although exercise has many other benefits.

2. Sweating in a sauna or steam room is effective at releasing toxins through the skin. At least fifteen to twenty minutes is necessary to achieve this objective. I recommend starting with one or two sessions per week.

3. If you do not tolerate the heat from a traditional sauna, infrared saunas are a good alternative. These achieve the same benefits in terms of detoxification but do not heat the air around the body. People who are intolerant of traditional saunas often do well with infrared saunas.

4. If you do not have access to any of these, it is also possible to use a bathtub at home. Fill the bathtub with hot water and immerse your body in it for at least fifteen minutes until you feel some sweat on your forehead. You may wish to put a quarter cup of bentonite clay into the water to prevent your body from absorbing any chemicals in the water through your skin.

## Keep Your Lymphatic System Healthy

The lymphatic system is part of the circulatory system, comprising a network of channels called lymphatic vessels that carry a clear fluid called lymph toward the heart. Keeping a healthy lymphatic system is important for the immune system as well as for removing toxins from the body. Unlike blood, the lymph fluid is not pumped by the heart but instead relies on muscular contraction and body movement to move the fluid appropriately.

1. Regular aerobic exercise is beneficial not only for cardiovascular health but also for lymphatic drainage.

2. More gentle physical activities such as yoga or tai chi are also effective.

3. Dry skin brushing can be a helpful way to move the lymph fluid throughout the body.

## Superfoods and Supplements for Daily Detoxification

1. One of the key elements that Ayurveda emphasizes for detoxification is healthy elimination through normal daily bowel movements. To facilitate this, drink adequate water and ensure that your diet contains plenty of fiber, especially soluble fiber, which can be obtained from fruits and vegetables.

2. Beets and especially beet greens are the richest food source of betaine, a natural phytochemical that supports healthy liver function. Incorporate beet greens into soup, salads, or smoothies.

3. Regularly consume cruciferous vegetables, which support Phase 2 liver pathways. These include bok choy, broccoli, brussels sprouts, cabbage, cauliflower, collards, kale, and turnips.

4. Ground flaxseeds are very beneficial because they contain lignans, powerful antioxidants that also help with hormone balance. It is important to grind flaxseeds, because otherwise they are just a fiber source, and your body cannot absorb the nutrients inside them. Ground flaxseeds are beneficial for detoxification and may reduce cancer risk as well. Eat one tablespoon daily.

5. Garlic has a variety of health benefits and aids detoxification by supporting the liver detox pathway of sulfate addition (or sulfation), as we discussed earlier. Other sulfur-rich foods that are helpful are eggs, onions, shallots, and leeks.

6. Turmeric has countless health benefits, as we discussed in Chapter 7. It is beneficial for detoxification because it supports Phase 2 liver detox enzymes.

7. Bentonite clay is a powerful adsorbent that binds toxins. It can be used in baths, clay masks, and other external uses. Warning: Do not take this supplement internally (except under strict supervision by a licensed practitioner) because it can cause severe constipation.

8. Chlorella is a type of algae that has been traditionally used for detoxification of heavy metals. While human studies are limited, one animal study did find reduced brain accumulation of mercury in rats fed chlorella powder while also ingesting mercury.[34] Chlorella is rich in other nutrients, including amino acids, vitamins, and minerals, and is well-tolerated. Add one to two teaspoons of chlorella powder to a smoothie. Please note that this may turn your stool a green color because of the deep green color of chlorella.

# CHAPTER 13
# THE PALEOVEDIC DETOX

Intensive detoxification programs are essential to help you achieve the next level of health. They are an important complement to the practices that promote regular, daily detoxification that we discussed in the preceding chapter. This section discusses my approach to more vigorous cleansing and reviews certain botanicals and nutritional supplements that can be used.

A specific three-week detoxification program that I call the Paleovedic Detox can be especially beneficial. This program helps you to eliminate commonly problematic foods, increase your intake of nutrient-dense healing foods, and begin the process of detoxification. The Paleovedic Detox helps you increase energy, reduce inflammation, burn fat, and begin to reverse disease.

There is an important reason why the program is twenty-one days and not longer or shorter. In Ayurvedic medicine, as we discussed earlier, there are three doshas and seven primary dhatus or tissues. It is believed that when you undertake a detox intentionally, one tissue level in each dosha is cleansed per day. Therefore, a time period of twenty-one days is ideal for all tissue levels in each of the doshas to be cleared. In Ayurveda, twenty-one days is an ideal amount of time for both physical and mental transformation.

## Paleovedic Detox

The goal of the Paleovedic Detox is to avoid the most allergenic foods and simplify your body's digestive processes to facilitate removal of toxins from your body and healing. Here are the detailed guidelines:

## Foods to Avoid

- All gluten and gluten-containing foods. These include grains like wheat, barley, rye, and spelt and processed foods that contain these grains, such as most breads, bagels, pasta, flour (white or whole wheat), and cereals.

- All dairy products. Examples include milk, yogurt, butter, cheese, ice cream, cottage cheese, or whey protein.
- Soy products. These include tofu, tempeh, soy milk, edamame, soy sauce, (which also contains gluten from wheat), and soy nuts.
- Corn. This includes fresh corn and all foods made from cornmeal or corn flour, such as polenta, popcorn, corn chips, and corn tacos.
- All "bad fats." Examples are hydrogenated oils, trans fatty acids, margarine, and vegetable seed oils such as corn oil, soybean oil, and vegetable oil. Also avoid all fried foods.
- Alcohol. While alcohol in moderation can be health-promoting, for the purposes of this detox, it is optimal to avoid alcohol so that your liver can potentially be engaged in processing other toxins.
- Caffeine. It is best to eliminate caffeine completely, but if for whatever reason you cannot completely eliminate this, try to reduce your caffeine intake as much as possible.
- All legumes except mung beans (used to make kitcheri as described below). This includes black beans, pinto beans, kidney beans, lentils, and so forth, and most important, peanuts (highly allergenic and actually a legume, not a nut).
- Sugar and artificial sweeteners. This includes white sugar, high-fructose corn syrup, candies, soda, and any product with added sugar, such as beverages, juices, jams, or spreads with added sugar.
- Conventionally grown meat, poultry, or eggs, or farm-raised fish.
- (Optional) Nightshade vegetables. If you have an autoimmune disease or suspect that you might have a reaction to nightshades, which include eggplant, tomatoes, bell peppers, chili peppers, white potatoes, and tomatillos, you can also eliminate this category of vegetables.

## Foods to Eat

- All grass-fed, organic, and/or pasture-raised meats and free-range poultry.
- Wild-caught oily fish, especially salmon, sardines, and mackerel.
- Organic or pastured eggs.
- A large number of vegetables (except corn); try to get at least twelve servings of vegetables per day. Make sure you include at least one cup

daily of cooked cruciferous vegetables to support healthy liver function (broccoli, brussels sprouts, cauliflower, cabbage, kale, bok choy, etc.).

- All fruits are okay except for canned, dried or processed fruits, or fruits with added sugar. Aim for at least two servings of fruit per day.
- Root vegetables. You may liberally eat root vegetables such as potatoes, sweet potatoes, beets, carrots, and so forth, as long as they are not processed—that is, no french fries or chips of any kind.
- Healthy fats. These include extra-virgin olive oil, coconut oil, flax seed oil, avocado oil, avocados, and nuts and seeds. Although many dairy products are healthy fats, I recommend avoiding them for the purpose of this cleanse, except for ghee or clarified butter.
- Fermented foods, such as sauerkraut, kimchi, coconut-milk yogurt, and kombucha. Aim for at least one type of fermented food each day.
- Bone broth, which is rich in minerals, amino acids, and gelatin, is very healing for the gut. Try to have bone broth at least four to five times each week.
- All nuts and seeds except peanuts. Choices include almonds, cashews, walnuts, pumpkin seeds, sunflower seeds, pecans, and so forth. Nut butters are acceptable as well.
- Consume at least one to two tablespoons of ground flaxseeds daily, which are beneficial for fiber content and intestinal detoxification. You can incorporate flaxseeds into smoothies or sprinkle them on top of salads or stir-fried vegetables.
- Spices. Try to consume a variety of spices every day, especially the spices discussed in Chapter 7. Other options for seasoning include lemon juice, lime juice, balsamic vinegar, tomato sauce or salsa, garlic, onions, and green onions. A good substitute for soy sauce is coconut-based alternative Coconut Secret Raw Coconut Aminos.
- (Optional) Kitcheri is a traditional Ayurvedic dish consisting of rice and mung beans that is very beneficial for detoxification. You may consume this up to once a day during the detox. I like a version of kitcheri known as masala kitcheri that incorporates healing spices. The recipe is in Appendix B.
- Gluten-free grains like white rice, quinoa, millet, wild rice, amaranth, buckwheat, teff, and arrowroot as well as products made from these grains are acceptable for occasional use as long as they are properly prepared and cooked and well-tolerated.

- Sweetener options. Stevia extract may be used without limitation. You can also use very small amounts of raw unfiltered honey, unrefined maple syrup, xylitol, erythritol, and fruit-based sweeteners such as monk fruit extract.
- Beverage options besides water include caffeine-free herbal tea and less than eight ounces per day of 100 percent fruit juice. Also, dairy-free soy-free milk alternatives such as almond milk, coconut milk, hemp milk, or rice milk are acceptable.

## Other Things to Do

- Hydration is very important. Drink six to eight glasses of purified water daily. Filtered tap water is best.
- Plan to get enough sleep every night so that you wake up feeling well-rested and energized (for most people, at least seven to eight hours). For ideas on how to improve your sleep habits, please refer to Chapter 10.
- Aim for thirty minutes of light to moderate aerobic exercise at least four to five times per week. This could include walking, light jogging, swimming, or exercise on gym equipment such as a stairmaster or elliptical machine.
- Practice a mind-body relaxation technique such as diaphragmatic breathing or meditation for at least fifteen minutes daily. This can be broken up into two eight-minute sessions or practiced in a single fifteen-minute session. For instructions and sample techniques, please see Chapter 11.
- Try to sweat in a sauna or steam room fifteen minutes, two to three times per week. Sweating enhances detoxification through the skin.
- If possible, try to have sex regularly (this takes your mind off of all the foods that you have given up during the cleanse, burns extra calories, increases oxygenation, and helps relieve stress).

## Supplements

Supplements can help support your body's detoxification pathways. It is best to take supplements under the supervision of a licensed practitioner. The recommendations listed here are general guidelines and need to be individualized for each person. If you experience any type of adverse reaction while you are taking a supplement, stop taking it immediately and consult with your practitioner; if you are not sure whether you are having an adverse reaction, stop taking the supplement until you get medical advice. You should start with a low dose and increase slowly. For detoxification support, there are various options to choose from:

- Metagenics UltraClear Plus pH—this is a product that contains a base of rice protein combined with vitamins, minerals, and other nutrients that support detoxification pathways. The recommended final dose to build up to is two scoops twice a day. As with all liver support, it's important to build up to the final dose gradually. Start with half a scoop or, if you are sensitive, a quarter of a scoop twice a day. Increase the dosage by half a scoop per day every three days until you achieve the final dose of two scoops twice a day. If at any point you get uncomfortable symptoms of any kind, reduce the dose to the level that does not cause any symptoms for you. For people who don't like to take pills, this is a liquid shake that can also serve as a meal replacement.
- Standard Process offers a variety of supplements that can be used to support detoxification. Their products are only sold through healthcare professionals, so find a practitioner in your area who works with these products (for advice about how to find a practitioner, see Chapter 15). Typical supplements I recommend during detoxification are Standard Process Livaplex and Standard Process SP Cleanse. The dose should be individualized, but with all supplements I recommend the "start low and go slow" approach. Liver support supplements can help your body release toxins, which can sometimes cause symptoms like headaches, gastrointestinal distress, and rashes. The way to minimize these reactions is to start slowly so that your body can get used to the detoxification process and clear toxins more gradually. Please work with a licensed professional to determine the correct dosages.
- Metagenics AdvaClear contains vitamins, minerals, and botanicals that support healthy detox pathways. The suggested dose is two tablets twice a day with food. You can either take this supplement on its own, or if you want to provide additional detoxification support for your body you can combine it with the Metagenics UltraClear Plus PH or Standard Process products.
- If you prefer not to take a supplement, another option is using herbal teas. These are less potent but usually well-tolerated, especially if you are

someone sensitive to supplements. Herbal teas that contain dandelion, milk thistle, or artichoke are good options. Good examples are Yogi Tea DeTox or Traditional Medicinals EveryDay Detox.

Ensure that you have at least one bowel movement daily. Proper elimination is essential during the detoxification because so many toxins are cleared through the stool. Ayurveda considers anything less frequent than one bowel movement per day to be constipation. If you are not eliminating daily, you may take either of the following supplements:

- Triphala 500 mg tablets—1 tablet daily at bedtime. Triphala—which means "three fruits" in Sanskrit—is a well-known Ayurvedic medicine that features equal parts of three dried fruits (haritaki, bibhitaki, and amalaki). Increase the dosage by one tablet every night to a maximum of four tablets until you are having at least one soft bowel movement daily. I like the brand Banyan Botanicals because they are certified organic and test their supplements for heavy metals (which sometimes contaminate Ayurvedic supplements). Triphala has powerful detoxification properties and can be an excellent adjunct during the cleanse even if you don't need it to stimulate bowel movements.
- An alternative is magnesium, which is available in various forms, such as magnesium citrate, magnesium oxide, or magnesium gycinate. Any form is acceptable. Most people find that magnesium at a dose of 400 to 800 mg per day is very helpful at promoting regular soft bowel movements. Too much magnesium can cause loose stools or diarrhea.
- Avoid laxatives like senna or cascara sagrada, which can be too strong and should only be used for short-term purposes only.

## Questions and Answers about the Detox

*How will I feel?*

I have seen a wide variety of responses from patients to this program. Some feel better than they have ever felt in their lives before, describing a profound increase in energy and vitality. Others feel some side effects or unpleasant symptoms as their body begins to release toxins that it has been holding on to for years or even decades. Possible symptoms include headaches, fatigue, aches and pains, upset stomach, rashes, sinus congestion, postnasal drip, and/or general malaise. If this is the case with you, my main advice to you would be this: be patient. Usually these symptoms gradually get better as the detox continues. Remember that this is a sign that your body is expelling toxins and that this is going to be very beneficial for you long-term. If the symptoms become too much, stop taking whichever supplement you are taking. Wait two days, and resume at a lower dose; increase to the highest dose that you can tolerate that does not cause adverse reactions. Every person is unique, and you have to determine what works for you.

*What happens if I "cheat"?*

I want to reassure you that it's okay if you are not perfect in following the diet and other recommendations. With that said, maximal benefit will likely result from adhering to the program as strictly as possible. Just do your best, and if for whatever reason you are not able to stick to the diet for a meal or two, it will not throw off the entire detox and invalidate any benefits—you will still find benefit from the program.

*How do I come off the detox and reintroduce foods?*

I recommend doing this gradually and introducing one major category of food every three days. Do not introduce more than one category of foods on the same day, because it makes it difficult to determine the cause of any reactions. For example, you may want to begin by reintroducing dairy products and observe how you feel the next couple of days, looking for any reactions. Possible signs that you might be sensitive to a food include gas, bloating, constipation or diarrhea, rashes, headaches, sleep changes, sinus congestion, postnasal drip, muscle stiffness, joint pains, or general malaise. If you are not sure whether you have had a reaction to a food category, consume more of the suspected foods to see if your reaction worsens. It is helpful to keep a food journal during this time to track your symptoms and help keep things organized.

When you are introducing a particular category, I suggest eating foods from that category at least two or even three times in that day to maximize the possibility that your body will manifest a reaction to it if you are indeed sensitive to that food. For example, if you are bringing back dairy products, you may want to have some yogurt, kefir, and butter on that day; if you are reintroducing corn, you could have popcorn, corn tacos, and polenta on the same day.

If you do not notice any symptoms for seventy-two hours after you reintroduce a food, then you can add that category of foods to your "OK list" and then move on to the next category. For example, if you reintroduce dairy on Monday and feel completely wonderful until Thursday morning, then you can assume that dairy is fine and reintroduce a different category on Thursday. You can continue to eat foods that have been previously reintroduced successfully, so in this example, you could still eat dairy on Thursday and then add another food. Your list of well-tolerated foods will be cumulative.

*How often should I do this detox?*

Ayurveda recommends some type of detoxification program during the change of seasons, for example, when winter changes to spring and spring changes to summer. Therefore, the ideal would be about four times per year. A minimum of twice a year would be beneficial for most people because of the continuous low-level exposure to toxins that all of us experience in our modern environment.

# CHAPTER 14

# HOW TO STAY HEALTHY—AVOIDING COMMON PITFALLS USING FOODS AND SUPPLEMENTS

The key in Ayurveda to staying healthy is having good digestion and a strong Agni, or digestive fire. Having a healthy gut flora is also fundamental to good health, as we discussed earlier. Keeping your Agni strong and your microbiome healthy with the strategies we discussed in earlier chapters will go a long way toward ensuring that you can maintain optimal wellness. This chapter discusses nutritional elements such as vitamins and minerals and includes a detailed discussion about supplements that can help to keep you healthy.

## Should I Take a Multivitamin?

This is one of the most common questions I hear from my patients. You might recall that when we were discussing the hormesis model of antioxidants in Chapter 7, I talked about a study showing no benefit in reducing risk of metabolic syndrome from long-term intake of antioxidant supplements.[1] The antioxidants tested in this study include vitamins such as vitamin C, vitamin D, beta-carotene, and minerals such as selenium. You might wonder why taking additional vitamins and minerals that are typically found in a multivitamin would not be beneficial to health, since most health authorities say that taking vitamins is good for you.

The reason is that the vitamins and minerals available in whole foods are much more complex than the vitamins and minerals in supplements. For example, the entire vitamin E complex includes four tocopherols, four tocotrienols, selenium, xanthine, lipositols, and other factors.[2] In contrast, what you will typically see in a standard multivitamin or vitamin supplement is just alpha-tocopherol, which can legally be labeled "Vitamin E" according to FDA standards. Thus, there really is a major difference between complete nutrients present in whole foods and the isolated constituents in supplements. It's not surprising that studies on the use of isolated antioxidants as supplements have shown harmful effects. The body simply is not used to receiving incomplete pieces of synthetic vitamins packaged in isolated supplements.

It does better with complete vitamin and mineral complexes in whole foods. Therefore, when partial components of vitamins are given as supplements, they do not have the same hormetic benefits on antioxidant status and, in fact, may cause other imbalances that could lead to adverse effects.

This is one reason I do not recommend vitamins or minerals to my patients, unless they are deficient in certain nutrients based on the results of laboratory testing. With that said, almost all the patients I test, even those with an impeccable diet, have some type of nutritional deficiency. I think this may have something to do with the depletion of soils, because plants only have as much nutrients as they can absorb from the soils that they are grown in. Research using data from the US Department of Agriculture has shown that today's produce, compared to identical produce from the mid-twentieth century, is significantly lower in calcium, phosphorus, iron, vitamin B2, and vitamin C, and probably lower in other nutrients as well.[3] New crop varieties engineered for rapid growth and changes in farming techniques, in addition to soil depletion, are likely responsible for these changes.

Other factors such as the stress of modern life and the toxins in our environment also increase the amount of nutrients that our bodies need and use every day. Illness can also increase your nutritional requirements. This combination of increased nutrient need and reduced availability of vitamins and minerals from our food is why most of my patients have some type of micronutrient deficiency.

Nutritional status and antioxidant status are critically important for good health. My approach is not to use supplements unless functional medicine testing identifies specific deficiencies and determines dosage guidelines for repletion. Based on that, I usually recommend whole-food supplements, which are supplements made from concentrated whole foods that are able to preserve the complexity of food-based nutrients. If you are not able to do nutritional testing, a whole-food multivitamin that is a blend of different foods, like Standard Process Catalyn GF or New Chapter multivitamins, are reasonable options.

## It Is Not Easy to Check Vitamin and Mineral Levels

Incidentally, it is not as easy as you might think to assess vitamin and mineral status. You might think that it is simply a matter of measuring blood levels of a particular vitamin, but it is not that straightforward. For example, with magnesium, the vast majority of your body's magnesium is intracellular, or within your cells. Very little is actually circulating in your blood. Therefore, measuring serum magnesium level is often not too helpful in evaluating magnesium status. The magnesium stores within your cells have to decline a great deal before the levels in the blood will begin to be affected; therefore, only late-stage magnesium deficiency will show up in your serum magnesium level. I like to check intracellular magnesium levels within the red blood cells, which offer a better indicator of true magnesium status.

## The Solution—Organic Acid Testing

Biochemistry testing using urine organic acids provides an accurate measure of vitamin levels. Organic acids are normal compounds that are made in the body through routine cellular processes that require vitamins and minerals. If the body does not have adequate levels of vitamins and minerals, it will be reflected in abnormal levels of organic acids. These markers help to individualize nutritional recommendations for each person.

Genetic factors, stresses, toxin levels, and environmental exposures all affect how much of each nutrient you need. In contrast, serum blood tests have a normal range for the entire population as a whole and do not take these differences into account. For example, someone with defects in genetic pathways affecting a process known as methylation may have a higher need for certain types of B vitamins. Someone dealing with a very stressful job may have a high need for certain other B vitamins. Another individual who is dealing with a mold problem at home and living in a big city with a lot of traffic may need higher levels of nutrients that support detoxification. Organic acid testing helps to determine the optimal nutritional requirements that you have at a certain point in time, given your unique biochemical status and all the internal and external stressors in your life.

Functional biochemistry testing using organic acids also enables me to track progress in correcting vitamin and mineral deficiencies. As with all things in the body, the balance is rather delicate, and supplementation may not be straightforward. I never simply prescribe a vitamin or mineral to a patient and have him or her take it long-term without tracking his or her levels. I want to ensure that the patient's body is getting the optimal level of nutrients, not too much or too little. A good example is vitamin D. Some patients get their levels up extremely quickly and in fact could develop a harmful excess of vitamin D if we do not take them off at the right time. Other patients have a very hard time raising their vitamin D level and require massive doses for a long period of time to bring their levels up.

## Vitamin D

Almost universally, my patients have some degree of vitamin D deficiency. Vitamin D, which is actually a hormone rather than a vitamin, has many important effects in the body and is critical for bone health, cancer prevention, immune system function, and cardiovascular health. It is important to measure your 25 hydroxy-vitamin D level (25-OH Vitamin D) to see where you stand:

| 25-OH Vitamin D Level | Classification |
|---|---|
| <29 | Low |
| 30–39 | Normal but suboptimal |
| 40–50 | Optimal |
| 51–99 | Only recommended for cancer patients |
| >100 | Potentially harmful |

With vitamin D, it is possible to make it from sun exposure, but you need substantial direct sunlight daily without sunscreen, which is hard to achieve. It is present in food sources like seafood, dairy products, and mushrooms, but not in large amounts. Therefore, most people require a supplement to boost their vitamin D levels.

I suggest you talk to your physician about checking your vitamin D levels. It is important to track your progress by rechecking the levels two to three months after supplementation. I have had patients who have rapidly attained levels that were too high and had to immediately stop taking it. Other patients have experienced side effects from excessive vitamin D, so it is not without risk.

## Vitamin $B_{12}$

In my experience, blood levels of vitamin $B_{12}$ are often not helpful in detecting vitamin $B_{12}$ deficiency. Even patients who have serum $B_{12}$ levels in the normal range can have symptoms such as neuropathy and related blood abnormalities such as anemia. Such symptoms and blood abnormalities often improve when vitamin $B_{12}$ is supplemented. The way that I determine the true need for vitamin $B_{12}$, and all vitamins and minerals, is through a functional medicine test measuring organic acids, as discussed above. For vitamin $B_{12}$, a key marker is urinary methylmalonic acid (MMA).

If only blood levels are available, I like to get patients in the upper half of the normal range. Food sources of vitamin $B_{12}$ include meat, poultry, fish, eggs, and dairy products. I have a low threshold for trying supplemental $B_{12}$ if a person has symptoms that seem like he or she might improve with $B_{12}$.

## Magnesium

Magnesium is a mineral that most of my patients are deficient in and that is sometimes hard to get adequately through food. Magnesium affects hundreds of metabolic and cellular processes and is one of the most vital minerals for overall health. Symptoms of low magnesium include fatigue, poor sleep, migraine headaches, muscle spasms, hair loss, constipation, anxiety, and thyroid problems.

Just how important is magnesium? Studies have shown that in hospitalized patients, magnesium deficiency *increases the risk of dying significantly* and prolongs hospital stay.[4] Most of these studies looked at blood levels of magnesium, which as I discussed earlier, can miss mild or moderate magnesium deficiency.

I would suggest having a red blood cell magnesium level checked by your physician. Get your levels into the upper half of the normal range defined by your laboratory. Reference ranges can vary, but a typical normal range is 4.0 to 6.1; in this example, you would want your level to be above 5.0.

To boost magnesium, consume plenty of magnesium-rich foods, such as green leafy vegetables, nuts, seafood, avocados, legumes, and (my favorite) dark chocolate—one of many reasons to have a small piece of dark chocolate every day.

Magnesium supplements are easily found, but there are significant differences in bioavailability or how much of the magnesium is absorbed. The main side effect of magnesium is diarrhea, which is a function of how much magnesium stays behind in your intestine after normal digestion and absorption. Magnesium draws water into your intestines, contributing to loose stools. The more bioavailable the magnesium is, the more is absorbed and the less stays in your intestinal tract to soften the stool. Magnesium oxide and sulfate have relatively lower bioavailability. However, if you suffer from constipation, these may be good options.

Magnesium gluconate, aspartate, lactate, and glycinate have higher bioavailability; magnesium citrate also is fairly well absorbed.[5] Transdermal magnesium oils and creams, which are absorbed directly through the skin, may be helpful in treating muscle cramps and spasms related to magnesium deficiency. They can be used by patients who cannot tolerate oral magnesium.

## Zinc

Zinc is a vital nutrient, important for immune function, cell growth, cell division, and wound healing. Many of my patients are low in zinc. A blood level of zinc is an acceptable way to assess levels—again, you want to be in the upper half of the normal range. Consume plenty of foods rich in zinc, such as green leafy vegetables, mushrooms, grass-fed meat, nuts, seeds (pumpkin seeds are loaded with zinc), seafood, legumes, and (yes it's true!) dark chocolate.

## Vitamin $K_2$

Vitamin $K_2$ is an important nutrient that can help reduce the risk of heart disease, improve bone health, promote healthy skin, prevent osteoporosis, and possibly protect against the development of cancer. It is distinct from vitamin $K_1$, which is found in leafy vegetables and primarily involved in blood clotting. Food sources of vitamin $K_2$ include meat, especially organ meats, as well as egg yolks, grass-fed butter and cheese, and fermented vegetables. For those who are adventurous, the richest food source of vitamin $K_2$ by far is *natto*, a fermented soybean product, which I enjoy, but some find revolting.

## Selenium

Selenium is a vital trace mineral that is important for thyroid hormone synthesis, immune function, antioxidant protection, and cancer and cardiovascular disease prevention. Selenium-rich foods include seafood, meat (especially organ meats), eggs, dairy products, and nuts. The richest food source of selenium is the Brazil nut; consuming two to three Brazil nuts daily will easily meet your daily requirements for selenium. Many Americans consume adequate amounts of selenium. Work with your functional medicine practitioner to assess your need for selenium.

## Omega-3 Fats

Maintaining a healthy omega-6 to omega-3 ratio of 4:1 or lower is very important, as we discussed in Chapter 3. It is possible to measure this ratio using specialized functional medicine lab testing. The last time I checked, my ratio was 3.4:1. The best way to achieve this is to decrease your intake of omega-6 fats and increase your intake of omega-3 fats. (For details on omega-3 and omega 6 fats, please refer to Chapter 3.)

Omega-3s are best derived from whole fish rather than from fish oil supplements. If you are able to eat fish at least three to four times per week or eat a pound per week of cold-water fatty fish, you do not need a fish oil supplement. If you don't eat fish, it may be beneficial to take a fish oil supplement.

## How to Choose a Fish Oil Supplement

When choosing a fish oil supplement, there are a few factors to keep in mind. First, you want to choose a brand that regularly tests for heavy metals, PCBs, and dioxins. Good quality brands state on their label that they regularly perform third-party testing for toxins. Secondly, look for products that are molecularly distilled, as these are more potent and lower in contaminants. Third, you want fish oil that has been derived from fish that are low in mercury, such as sardines, anchovies, and salmon.

Norwegian brands such as Nordic Naturals or Carlson meet these criteria. Vital Choice is a company that sells sustainably harvested wild Alaskan salmon in both food and supplement form; their wild salmon oil is an excellent option. Jarrow Formulas also offers a quality product that meets these criteria and is less expensive than some of the other brands.

Ideally, you want fish oil that is processed at cold temperatures. Fermented cod liver oil is one product that has distinct advantages in this category. It is processed at cold temperatures, prepared in a traditional fermentation process, and rich in vitamins A and D in addition to containing omega-3 fatty acids. It is also rich in vitamin $K_2$, an important vitamin for bone health and cardiac health that is not present in many foods. Also, fermented cod liver oil is more like a food than a supplement, so it's safe for long-term use—unlike fish oil supplements, which should be used for a specific time period determined by you and your practitioner.

If you are vegetarian or vegan, you can opt for algae-based omega-3 supplements. They contain more DHA than EPA, but both of these omega-3 fatty acids are beneficial. The main downside is cost, as the supplements tend to be expensive.

## What about Krill Oil?

Krill are tiny shrimp-like creatures that exist by the billions in the ocean. As with fish, they eat plankton, which are the source of omega-3 fatty acids. A relatively new product, krill oil does not have as much research support behind it as fish oil. There are only a handful of studies of krill oil, and most of them have been funded by krill oil companies, raising questions about conflict of interest. In contrast, there is a substantial research literature on the benefits of fish oil. For example, fish oil has been proven to reduce sudden death in people with heart disease,[6] whereas krill oil has not been studied.

The omega-3 content of krill oil tends to be relatively lower compared to the omega-3 content of fish oil. Certain antioxidants in krill oil, such as astaxanthin, may have other benefits, but we don't have research on this. In addition, there are potential adverse environmental impacts from the way that krill oil is made. Therefore, although this could change based on future research, I don't recommend krill oil over fish oil.

## How to Store and Take Fish Oil

For optimal absorption, take fish oil supplements with a meal that contains some fat. Don't take fish oil on an empty stomach. To prevent fish oil from turning rancid, store it in your freezer. This also eliminates problems with "fishy burps" after taking fish oil. With fermented cod liver oil, there is no need to store it in the freezer as it is shelf-stable.

## Food Is Foundational

It is best to get most of your vitamins, minerals, and other nutrients from food. However, soil depletion and changes in our crop varieties and farming practices have reduced the nutritional content of our food. If you incorporate the Paleovedic Diet and consume plenty of whole foods, you will still have a good nutritional foundation. Functional medicine testing can help identify specific nutrient deficiencies, which can then be addressed with foods or targeted supplements. Whole-food supplements are generally preferable to isolated vitamins and minerals and can help fill gaps in your nutritional status.

# CHAPTER 15

# PUTTING IT ALL TOGETHER—YOUR CUSTOMIZED FOOD PLAN

In this chapter, we integrate all the information about diet from throughout the book to create your individual customized dietary plan. I tell you exactly what you can eat, breaking it down into foods you should eat daily, occasionally (four to five times per week), and rarely (one time or less a week). I also cover what foods you should avoid eating.

## My Philosophy on Food

Before I get into the specific recommendations, I want to review my general philosophy about diet. First, Ayurvedic medicine reminds us that we should "eat to live" and not "live to eat." While it is critical to plan meals carefully and try to eat as well as you can, it is important not to become fanatical about eating the perfect food all the time. There is a condition now known as orthorexia, which describes an obsession with eating only "proper" foods; unwarranted negative feelings such as guilt and regret may occur when one deviates from this regimen.

Some of my patients have described their challenges with this syndrome. Especially in the San Francisco Bay Area, it is very easy to follow a relatively clean diet. However, this can be taken to an extreme, and people can struggle with this when they become overly rigid about the types of foods they can eat. Some patients have reported having to cook and prepare all of their meals by themselves and being unable to eat at a restaurant or even at a friend's house, which is also very isolating socially. Others talk about being paralyzed while shopping for groceries because it is impossible to be 100 percent perfect with every single food that you buy at a grocery store; sometimes even certified organic foods have food additives.

With most people, I recommend the 90:10 rule. This means that 90 percent of the time you stick to your prescribed diet and do the best that you can to eat healthy. Ten percent of the time, which translates to once or a maximum of twice per week, you can give yourself a treat and consume foods that are not a part of your usual diet—typically this is when you might go out to a restaurant for a meal and have less control over all the ingredients that go into your meal anyway. When working with patients whose digestive system is imbalanced, I am usually more strict while we are improving the overall function of their digestive tract. However, once things are stable, as long as they are not struggling with major gastrointestinal issues or other serious food allergies, they should be able to broaden and expand their diet. If they cannot tolerate this, something may not be quite right with their digestion.

Ayurveda believes that if you have a strong Agni, or digestive fire, you should be able to eat a wide range of foods and effectively process them, even if this includes some foods that are harder to digest. To me, the modern equivalent of this is having a healthy microbiome, adequate digestive enzymes, and good gut motility, all hallmarks of good digestion. If your digestive system is in good shape, you should be able to handle a variety of foods and have no issues with more challenging foods consumed occasionally while following the 90:10 rule.

The other aspect about food that is very important is eating your food in a mindful, unhurried state. Try not to eat when you are extremely rushed or stressed out. Always try to sit down while eating, and do not stand up and eat (this is a no-no in Ayurveda). Minimize distractions such as television, Internet, and the use of other screens. Chewing your food thoroughly and paying attention to your meal will make you less likely to overeat.

If possible, try to enjoy at least one meal each day sitting down together with family or friends, not only for the social connection but because studies suggest that this helps control portion size. Many people eat for psychological reasons such as loneliness, anxiety, and emotional stress; if you find you are reaching for food for one of these reasons and not due to genuine hunger, seek out an alternative outlet.

Now that we have talked about a healthy approach to food, let us discuss specific dietary recommendations. You may be curious about my diet, so let me start by describing that in the following section.

## The Doctor's Diet

For many years after I resumed eating meat, I followed a moderate-carbohydrate diet, always avoiding sugar, flour, vegetable oils, and most sweets.

Currently, my diet has evolved to be a low-carbohydrate diet, which I don't recommend for everyone—but I know it works well for me. I tolerate legumes quite well, possibly due to my Indian heritage, and therefore incorporate properly cooked and prepared legumes regularly. In fact, when I tried eliminating legumes, I actually felt worse.

My diet is rich in plant-based nutrients from vegetables of all colors and high in protein from eggs, meat, and seafood. I eat root vegetables such as sweet potatoes, potatoes, carrots, beets, cassava daily. My diet also includes fermented full-fat dairy products, pickled vegetables, two servings of fruit each day, plenty of spices, green tea, dark chocolate, and the occasional indulgence in my all-time favorite dessert, tiramisu (following the 90:10 rule). For vitamin $K_2$, I occasionally eat *natto*, a fermented Japanese soybean dish that was initially nauseating but has become an acquired taste. People tend to have strong feelings about the taste of *natto*, with some considering it a delicacy and others describing it as vile—I suggest you try it. It has more vitamin $K_2$ by orders of magnitude than any other food on the planet (more about vitamin $K_2$ in Chapter 14), but make sure to get organic, non-GMO *natto*. I avoid soy from other sources.

I also feel best when I incorporate Ayurvedic nutrition guidelines for my vata body type—eating more cooked vegetables and minimizing salads and raw foods, making extensive use of spices, and consuming a great deal of oils and fats, including what my friends call "unholy" amounts of ghee. Other fats in my diet that I eat every day are extra virgin olive oil, coconut oil, avocados, and nuts and seeds.

Now let us go into the details of the Paleovedic Diet.

## Foods to Avoid in the Paleovedic Diet:

- **Refined grains, especially white flour, wheat flour (or whole wheat flour).** Refined grains are made by pulverizing whole grains and removing the most nutritious components of grains, such as the bran and the endosperm. What's left is the calorie-rich, nutrient-poor staple of the Western diet—flour. Moreover, the intense heat and pressure required for industrial processing of grains probably creates other toxins. Scientists have reviewed some intriguing experiments with refined grains. In one peculiar study, laboratory rats were fed either their usual diet, cornflakes, or the cardboard box the cornflakes came in—the control group lived normally, while all the rats fed the cornflakes actually died before the cardboard-eating rats started dying.[1] Other studies have documented the harmful health effects from refined grains.

- **Vegetable seed oils.** These include all vegetable oils made from industrial processing, such as soybean oil, corn oil, canola oil, safflower oil, cottonseed oil, and a few others. The only healthy vegetable oils are olive oil and coconut oil. Red palm oil is nutritious but not recommended unless concerns about environmental sustainability are specifically addressed.

- **Trans fats.** Trans fats are made by hydrogenating vegetable oils to make them solid at room temperature. It is well-known now that trans fats promote inflammation and have a strong connection with heart disease. Even large food manufacturers are removing trans fats from their products. Avoid any food that contains hydrogenated or partially hydrogenated oils.

- **Refined sugar.** Added sugar, especially white sugar, worsens numerous metabolic markers, promotes inflammation, and has been associated with obesity, type 2 diabetes, and heart disease.

## Foods to Eat Every Day:

- **Organic or pastured eggs,** including the yolks (which are the most nutritious part). You may eat up to two eggs with the yolks every day.
- **Vegetables**, at least twelve servings per day. Vegetables are far and away the most important part of your diet. The phytochemicals and nutrients in vegetables are your primary defense against disease. Make sure you include plenty of nutrient-dense leafy green vegetables every day. Also frequently incorporate cruciferous vegetables, which protect against cancer and support healthy liver function (broccoli, brussels sprouts, cauliflower, cabbage, kale, bok choy, etc.).

- **Fruits**, up to two servings every day. Fruits are a great source of phytochemicals (refer to Chapter 4 guidelines about which fruits are most nutrient-dense). Because fruit is much higher in sugar than vegetables, I recommend limiting it to two servings per day for most people.
- **Root vegetables.** You may liberally eat root vegetables such as potatoes, sweet potatoes, beets, carrots, and so forth.
- **Healthy fats.** These include extra-virgin olive oil, coconut oil, avocados, grass-fed butter, and ghee. Coconut oil is especially beneficial, and I recommend that people try to eat one to two tablespoons daily. Coconut oil contains beneficial fats known as medium chain triglycerides that can inhibit the growth of harmful gut microbes, improve lipid profiles, promote weight loss, improve neurological function, and possibly protect against heart disease.[2] If you find that extra-virgin coconut oil has too strong of a coconut flavor, you can use expeller-pressed coconut oil, which is very mild and does not impart a strong flavor. Both forms are good, and we use both types of coconut oil at home. Flaxseed oil and hemp seed oil are good options for occasional use but should never be heated.
- **Other protein sources.** This could include organic, grass-fed meat or wild-caught seafood (see below) or if you are vegetarian, legumes, eggs, dairy products, and so forth.
- **Fermented and/or pickled vegetables.** I encourage daily consumption of fermented vegetables, because they are rich in probiotics and healthy acids. Sauerkraut is an excellent option. Your only memory of sauerkraut might be a pale, tasteless topping that you put on hot dogs. These days, a variety of delicious options with different flavors and various combinations of vegetables are available. Experiment with different brands to see what you like. Choose a brand that is prepared in a traditional manner and does not contain preservatives like sodium benzoate. It is also not difficult to make your own sauerkraut or other pickled vegetables at home—for detailed instructions, please visit my website.
- **Spices.** All spices are acceptable, especially the ones discussed in Chapter 7.

## Foods to Eat Frequently for All People, at least Four to Five Days per Week

- **Meat and poultry.** Grass-fed, organic, and/or pasture-raised meats and free-range poultry, including organ meats such as liver, at least once per week.
- **Fish**. Wild-caught oily fish, especially salmon, sardines, anchovies, and mackerel, for a total of a pound per week.
- **Bone broth** is rich in minerals, amino acids, and gelatin, which are all very healing for the gut.
- **Sprouts** such as clover, alfalfa, or broccoli sprouts offer a cornucopia of different nutrients and phytochemicals. Consuming them as often as you can would be highly beneficial. Bean sprouts are less nutrient-dense.
- **Tea**. Green, black, or white tea are all great sources of antioxidants and other phytochemicals. If you prefer, coffee is an acceptable alternative (preferably with full-fat cream). Another benefit of tea is that it provides an astringent taste according to Ayurveda, which as we discussed is often missing from modern diets.
- **Chocolate**. Aim for a minimum of 70 percent cocoa. Dark chocolate contains magnesium and zinc and is a rich source of polyphenols, which are beneficial for cardiovascular health and antioxidant status. Consume up to two ounces per day.
- **Fermented cod liver oil** (FCLO) is beneficial if you are not able to eat the recommended one pound of fish per week (or even if you are!). It is processed at cold temperatures, prepared in a traditional fermentation process, and rich in vitamins A and D in addition to containing omega-3 fatty acids. It is rich in vitamin $K_2$, which is important for cardiovascular health. Because this is a food, it is safe for long-term use, unlike fish oil supplements. It is available in either capsule or liquid form—I enjoy the cinnamon flavor FCLO from Green Pastures.
- **Seasonings**. Make liberal use of spices wherever you can! Other seasonings that are beneficial for digestion include apple cider vinegar, lemon juice, lime juice, balsamic vinegar, and green onions. A good substitute for soy sauce that I use is coconut-based alternative Coconut Secret Raw Coconut Aminos.
- **Beets.** Both the roots and the greens are incredibly nutritious. Beet greens, the leafy tops of beets, are the richest food source of betaine

(also known as trimethylglycine), which helps your body to detoxify by supporting methylation and Phase 2 liver detox pathways. Beet greens are one of the most powerful unheralded superfoods that can aid in detoxification. If you have a history of oxalate kidney stones, use caution with beets as they are high in oxalates.

- **Pickled ginger.** Ginger has an astonishing array of health benefits, and is especially good quieting inflammation, which is the root cause of most modern diseases. In pickled form, it has the additional benefits of a fermented food. Therefore, I recommend that you try to consume pickled ginger daily. You might know pickled ginger from sushi restaurants. While this is available in Asian markets, it usually has synthetic food dye to give it that familiar pink color. Natural markets typically have pickled ginger without artificial colors or preservatives. As a condiment, enjoy two or three pieces with meals as often as you like. There is no restriction for vata and kapha body types, who will benefit from the warming, stimulating properties of ginger. Pitta types should only have it occasionally because excess ginger can be excessively heating for them.

## Foods to Eat Frequently for Some People, up to Four to Five Days per Week

These are gray-area foods that some people do not tolerate but others thrive on. You can consume these foods frequently if you tolerate them well.

- **Dairy products.** I recommend only full-fat dairy products like yogurt, kefir, and cheese. Avoid low-fat dairy products because of increased risk of health problems as we discussed in the text. Butter and ghee are also excellent options.
- **Legumes**. This includes all types of beans, lentils, dhal, chickpeas, and other legumes except peanuts. Legumes should be properly prepared by soaking overnight, sprouting, and/or fermenting before they are cooked.
- **All nuts and seeds except peanuts.** Choices include almonds, cashews, walnuts, pumpkin seeds, sunflower seeds, ground flaxseeds, and so forth. Macadamia nuts and almonds are excellent choices because they are low in omega-6 fats (for details about the omega-6 content of nuts

and seeds, please refer to Chapter 3). Nut butters are acceptable as well. If you have difficulty digesting nuts, you can soak or sprout them.

- **Gluten-free grains** like white rice, quinoa, millet, wild rice, amaranth, buckwheat, teff, and arrowroot as well as products made from these grains are acceptable if you tolerate them well. Ayurveda does not recommend brown rice because it is difficult to digest.

## Foods to Eat Rarely (Once a Week or Less Frequently)

- **Corn.** The great majority of corn in this country is genetically modified, nutrient-poor, and excessively high in carbohydrates and sugar. Typically corn is processed heavily before entering the food supply. An occasional corn taco made from organic stone-ground whole cornmeal would be acceptable.
- **Soy.** The only type of soy that I recommend eating is fermented soy like *natto* (an incredible source of vitamin $K_2$) or miso. If you can tolerate *natto*, you only need to eat it once or twice per week to get its health benefits. Technically, tofu and tempeh are also fermented, but I do not recommend regular consumption unless you are vegetarian.
- **Peanuts**. One of my Ayurvedic teachers used to say "peanuts are poison." While Ayurveda has a favorable view of most nuts and seeds, it has a decidedly negative attitude toward peanuts (which are legumes and not really nuts anyway). Peanuts are highly allergenic, are often genetically modified, and have a less favorable fatty-acid profile than other nuts.
- **Sweeteners**. Occasional sweets made with natural sweeteners like raw honey, molasses, maple syrup, or stevia are acceptable. Avoid white sugar and artificial sweeteners such as aspartame, sucralose (Splenda), or acesulfame potassium, because these actually promote weight gain, negatively affect your microbiome, and have other harmful effects.

## Tailor Your Diet According to Your Ayurvedic Body Type

Use your Ayurvedic body type to further customize and individualize your optimal diet. To determine your body type and review Ayurvedic guidelines for tailoring your diet accordingly, please see Chapter 6.

## How Much to Eat

I do not believe in recommending a certain number of calories for each person. The "calories in/calories out" model of obesity has been clearly disproven. What really matters is the quality of the food that you are consuming. Calorie requirements vary widely based on genetics, metabolism, activity level, and other factors.

Ayurveda does not recommend tracking calories, and I strongly agree with this approach. The important recommendation is to eat until you are about two-thirds full. To use a simple example, if three portions of food would make you full, then eat two portions. It is important to learn to pay attention to signals of satiety and fullness, if you are not doing so already. Ayurveda does offer general guidelines for portion sizes.

## Portion Size for Meals

- Two handfuls of non-starchy vegetables per meal—the amount you would get if you cupped your hands and fingers together. This is the most important part of your diet and should be the foundation of every meal.
- One handful of starchy vegetables like root vegetables (sweet potatoes, potatoes, carrots, etc.) or healthy grains like white rice per meal.
- One palm-size portion of protein like meat, fish, or legumes, equivalent approximately to the surface area and thickness of your palm.
- Good fats such as ghee, coconut oil, and olive oil may be incorporated liberally depending on your body type—no restrictions for vata, moderate intake for pitta, and minimal or reduced intake for kapha.

## Last Words on Diet

I hope that you have a clear idea now about the diet that's optimal for you. Remember that it might change over time depending on changes in body composition, health status, fitness goals, and other factors. Ayurveda believes that your optimal diet is something fluid that can change depending on life circumstances.

Ultimately, eating nutrient-dense whole foods is the essence of the Paleovedic Diet. Adding in powerful healing spices, using Ayurveda to customize your diet, and incorporating foods and other elements that support detoxification are all critical elements that can help you take your health to the next level.

## Next Steps—Find a Practitioner to Work with

If you have incorporated the suggestions in this book but are still having health issues, it may be beneficial to work with a functional medicine practitioner. Functional medicine is the branch of integrative medicine that uses specialized lab testing to evaluate and optimize the function of various organ systems. Let's discuss how to find local functional medicine practitioners to work with.

There are three websites that can be helpful. First, the Institute for Functional Medicine is a national organization that provides training and educational programs for licensed practitioners in functional medicine. They have a website where you can search for practitioners who have completed their training programs: www.functionalmedicine.org/practitioner_search.aspx.

Another helpful website is the Paleo Physicians Network. This database, started by Loren Cordain and Robb Wolf, features practitioners who are familiar with the Paleo diet and often also practitioners of functional or integrative medicine. It includes physicians, acupuncturists, chiropractors, and other licensed health professionals. For more information, visit www.paleophysiciansnetwork.com.

Finally, a similar site that also features practitioners who are in the primal/ancestral space is www.primaldocs.com.

## Conclusion

Medicine is changing. I believe that integrative medicine, which incorporates alternative and conventional medicine, will be the medicine of the future. Combining safe and effective evidence-based complementary therapies with conventional medicine can help improve outcomes and lower costs. In a medical landscape with exorbitant costs, integrative medicine can offer low-cost tools to empower people to take a proactive approach to health.

The Paleovedic Diet is integrative medicine in action, bringing together the seemingly opposed worlds of ancient wisdom and modern science to create a comprehensive road map for wellness. I hope you will use the principles in this book to create your own customized diet and lifestyle plan for optimal health. My highest wish is that this book helps you to achieve spectacular health and vitality and to feel better than you have ever felt before. If enough people make positive healthy changes, we can alter our collective trajectory and begin to reverse our modern epidemics of obesity and chronic disease. I thank you, dear reader, for undertaking this journey—together we can transform our bodies and minds and our societies.

# APPENDIX A

# MENU PLAN FOR THE PALEOVEDIC DETOX BY SHARON MEYER

## 14-Day Menu

### Day 1

*Breakfast*

**Egg Muffins**

*Lunch*

**Ceviche**

*Dinner*

**Kerala Beef Liver Fry with Malabar Rice**

### Day 2

*Breakfast*

**Chicken Apple Sausage with Grilled Tomatoes**

*Lunch*

**Salmon Cakes on Mixed Greens with Smoky Lemon Vinaigrette**

*Dinner*

**Thai Pumpkin Soup**

### Day 3

*Breakfast*

**Masala Kitcheri**

*Lunch*

**Asian Steak Salad**

*Dinner*

**Stir-fried Beef and Broccoli**

### Day 4

*Breakfast*

**Poached Eggs over Spinach with Baked Pears**

*Lunch*

**Herby Chicken Patties on Malabar Rice**

*Dinner*

**Mushrooms and Shrimp in Saffron Coconut Curry Broth**

### Day 5

*Breakfast*

**Scrambled Eggs with Roasted Vegetables**

*Lunch*

**Crab with Avocado and Ginger**

*Dinner*

**Roast Lamb with Roasted Garlic Broccoli**

### Day 6

*Breakfast*

**Vegetable Omelet with Salsa**

*Lunch*

**Roasted Rosemary Chicken with a Green Salad**

*Dinner*

**Roasted Salmon with Salsa**

### Day 7

*Breakfast*

**Crust-less Quiche**

*Lunch*

**Salad with Chicken Apple Sausage**

*Dinner*

**Cioppino**

### Day 8

*Breakfast*

**Baked Eggs in Tomato Sauce**

*Lunch*

**Roasted Asparagus Soup**

*Dinner*

**Chicken Skewers with Artichoke and Lemon Pesto and Stir-fried Vegetables**

### Day 9

*Breakfast*

**Omelet with Crab and Avocado**

*Lunch*

**Buffalo Burgers with Mixed Salad Greens and Citrus Vinaigrette**

*Dinner*

**Halibut Parcels with Chives and Rosemary Roasted Sweet Potatoes**

### Day 10

*Breakfast*

**Baked Apples with Cilantro Cashew Cream**

*Lunch*

**Coconut Egg Curry over Rice Pilaf**

*Dinner*

**Lamb Kofta Topped with Baba Ganoush, Sliced Tomatoes, and Olives**

### Day 11

*Breakfast*

**Crust-less Quiche**

*Lunch*

**Salad with Chicken-Apple Sausage and Lemon Vinaigrette**

*Dinner*

**Tea-poached Salmon with Herby Pesto and Mock Mashed Potatoes**

### Day 12

*Breakfast*

**Egg Muffins**

*Lunch*

**Pork Satay with Brussels Sprouts**

*Dinner*

**Coconut Chicken and Red Cabbage with Apple and Cranberries**

### Day 13

*Breakfast*

**Congee with Added Egg**

*Lunch*

**Avocado with Shredded Crab**

*Dinner*

**Boboti with a Green Salad**

### Day 14

*Breakfast*

**Masala Kitcheri**

*Lunch*

**Tuna with Homemade Mayonnaise on a Green Salad**

*Dinner*

**Chili Topped with Cilantro Cashew Cream**

# APPENDIX B
# PALEOVEDIC RECIPES BY SHARON MEYER

This section contains recipes from the following categories—broths and soups, snacks and dips, appetizers, entrées, vegetables, and desserts. In general, the recipes do not contain gluten, wheat, corn, or dairy products. Vegetarians may substitute tofu or tempeh for meat ingredients when appropriate. I do include dessert on the menu every few days—this is optional, but if you consume it in small portions, there should not be any issue. All recipes are by Sharon Meyer unless otherwise credited.

## Broths and Soups

As you read in the Introduction, bone broths played a vital role in my recovery from illness and are therefore dear to my heart. Properly prepared meat and bone broths are extremely nutritious, containing the minerals of bone, cartilage, marrow, and vegetables as electrolytes in a form that is easy to assimilate. Acidic wine or vinegar added during cooking helps to draw minerals such as calcium, magnesium, and potassium into the broth.

# Chicken Bone Broth

2 chicken carcasses, or

1 whole chicken cut into portions, or 3 chicken backs and package of chicken feet, or Combination of all—(I like adding the chicken feet for wonderful gelatin)

4 quarts water

1 whole garlic head, quartered

1 whole onion, roughly chopped

2 carrots, roughly chopped

4 sticks celery, chopped

1 teaspoon peppercorns

1 teaspoon salt

3 bay leaves

1 bunch thyme or oregano (optional)

3 tablespoons vinegar

Put all the ingredients into a large stainless steel soup pot and let stand for 30 minutes.

Bring to a boil, then turn down the heat and simmer for 8–24 hours, or until the bones disintegrate when pressed with a fork. Another option is a lead-free slow cooker or Instant Pot pressure cooker; use the slow setting cook for 12–24 hours. Once the broth is done, pour it through a strainer. Keep the chicken pieces for coconut curry, mayonnaise chicken, or chicken lettuce cups.

Pour the broth into containers (I use mason jars). Refrigerate. After a few hours the fat will have congealed; remove it and seal your jars (don't fill all the way to the top) and freeze.

# Beef Bone Broth

4–5 pounds beef bones—knuckle, marrow, shin, and/or meatier neck parts
4–5 quarts water
1 whole garlic head, quartered
1–2 whole onions, roughly chopped
2 carrots (organic), roughly chopped
4 sticks celery, chopped
1 teaspoon peppercorns
1 teaspoon salt
1 bay leaf
1 bunch thyme or oregano (optional)
3 tablespoons vinegar
Salt and pepper
2 medium leeks, washed (keeping the root end intact, cut the leek in half lengthwise; give it a quarter turn, and then slice lengthwise again, keeping the root end intact—fan out the leaves and rinse out the sand and grit)

Put all the ingredients into a large stainless steel soup pot or lead-free slow cooker and let stand for 30 minutes.

If using a stock pot, bring to a boil, and then turn down to a simmer. In a slow cooker set to cook on low.

Simmer for 12–24 hours.

Once the broth is done, remove the bones using tongs, then pour broth through a strainer. Pour the broth into containers (I use mason jars). Refrigerate. After a few hours the fat will have congealed; remove it and seal your jars (don't fill all the way to the top) and freeze.

# Kerala Beef Liver Fry

1 pound beef liver, washed, drained, and chopped into 1-inch pieces
2 tablespoons expeller-pressed coconut oil
½ teaspoon turmeric powder
¼ teaspoon red chili powder
¼ teaspoon sea salt
¼ teaspoon fennel seeds
3-inch piece ginger, finely chopped
15 medium curry leaves, chopped or blended into small pieces
6 medium shallots, finely chopped
3 ounces shredded coconut (available frozen)
1 teaspoon ground black pepper
Chopped cilantro, for garnish

In a pressure cooker combine the cut beef liver, 1 tablespoon of coconut oil, turmeric powder, red chili powder, and salt. Stir well to distribute the spices evenly.

Cook on medium in a pressure cooker (with the pressure regulator on top) until you hear 2 whistles, and then turn the stove off, leaving the meat in the pressure cooker as it cools. If you are using a programmable electric pressure cooker, cook for about 15 minutes in the standard-setting, or using the "Beef" option.

In a skillet or cast-iron pan heat the remaining 1 tablespoon of coconut oil. When the oil is hot reduce the stove top to medium and fry the fennel seeds until they become fragrant. Then add the finely chopped ginger and fry until it becomes golden brown. Next add the curry leaves and cook for another minute. Then add the shallots and cook until they turn translucent. Finally, add the shredded coconut and black pepper.

Transfer the cooked liver into the skillet and cook on high while stirring well until any residual water evaporates.

After a few minutes, when the water has evaporated, remove from heat and garnish with chopped cilantro. Serve immediately.

*(recipe by Aiswarya Palanisamy)*

# Masala Kitcheri

1 cup uncooked white basmati rice
¼ cup split yellow mung dal
4 teaspoons ghee
1 teaspoon cumin seeds
1 piece (small stick) or ¼ teaspoon cinnamon
4 cloves
½ teaspoon black peppercorns
6 medium curry leaves
½ cup onions, finely chopped
¼ teaspoon ginger powder
1 clove garlic, finely minced
½ cup carrots, chopped into half-inch pieces
¼ teaspoon turmeric powder
½ teaspoon coriander powder
4 cups water
1 teaspoon salt

Soak the rice and yellow mung dal mixture in water for at least 30 minutes. Drain well and keep this aside. Heat ghee in a pressure cooker or stainless steel pot and add the cumin seeds. When it sizzles add the cinnamon, cloves, black peppercorns, and curry leaves. Now add the onions and sauté them for about 1 minute. Once the onions become translucent, add the ginger and garlic and sauté for 2 more minutes. Add the chopped carrots and cook for 1 minute. Then, add the remaining spices and mix well. Mix in the drained rice and dal mixture and stir well. Add water and salt and bring to a boil. Close the pressure cooker and cook on high heat until 3–4 whistles have elapsed. If you are using a pot on the stove top, ensure that the water level is about 2 inches above the top of the contents, and cook on low heat, stirring occasionally, until most of the water is absorbed—usually about 30 minutes. Serve while hot.

*(recipe by Aiswarya Palanisamy)*

## Mushrooms and Shrimp in Saffron Coconut Curry Broth

1 teaspoon saffron strands
4 tablespoons olive oil or coconut oil
1 onion, finely chopped
2 cups shitake mushrooms, roughly chopped
1 red pepper, deseeded and roughly chopped
1-inch long piece ginger, finely chopped
3 cloves garlic, crushed
1 tablespoon curry powder
1 teaspoon ground cumin
2 tablespoons Thai fish sauce
2 cups chicken or vegetable broth
1 (14-ounce) can regular coconut milk
1 pound of shrimp (cleaned) or salad shrimp
1 bunch of Swiss chard, washed and finely chopped
Salt and pepper

Put 1 teaspoon of saffron strands in 1 tablespoon of hot water and let stand for 15 minutes while you prepare the rest of the recipe.

In a Dutch oven add 4 tablespoons of olive oil or coconut oil, chopped onion, mushrooms, red pepper, and ginger and sauté for about 5–6 minutes or until the onions are translucent. Then add garlic, curry powder, cumin, Thai fish sauce, vegetable or chicken broth, coconut milk, and saffron in water and simmer for 10 minutes. Add the shrimp and finely chopped Swiss chard. Season with salt and pepper.

# Roasted Asparagus Soup

3 pounds of asparagus, ends removed, cut in half

2 large leeks (see instructions on how to wash under "Beef Bone Broth" page 222)

⅓ cup of olive oil

1 teaspoon of salt

1 teaspoon of pepper

1 clove of garlic minced

4 cups of chicken or vegetable stock

1 teaspoon of salt

1 teaspoon of pepper

1 tablespoon of fresh parsley

Place two baking sheets in the oven and preheat to 450 degrees.

In a large mixing bowl add the asparagus, leeks, oil, salt, and pepper. Mix well making sure the vegetables are well coated.

Place them on the hot baking sheets and roast for about 45 minutes until the asparagus is soft. You may have to stir occasionally to get an even roast.

Remove the vegetables from the baking sheets and cool. Blend ½ the vegetables, garlic, ½ the stock, and parsley in a blender or food processor. Pour the soup into a pot and do the same with the other ½ of the ingredients.

Gently heat the soup and if it's too thick add more broth.

# Thai Pumpkin Soup

2 tablespoons olive oil

2 tablespoons Thai red curry paste

1 stalk of lemongrass, finely chopped

2 cloves garlic, crushed

1 knob ginger, crushed

1 (14-ounce) can regular coconut milk

2–3 small pumpkins or any other squashes, peeled, seeded, and cut into chunks

2 tablespoons fish sauce

1 tablespoon coconut sugar

2 tablespoons lime juice

2 cups of chicken or vegetable broth

Heat the oil in a large saucepan or Dutch oven. Add the curry paste and cook for 1 minute; add lemongrass, garlic, and ginger and cook for 1 minute—keep stirring to prevent from sticking.

Add all the ingredients and bring to a boil, reduce the heat, and let simmer for 20–25 minutes before pureeing.

# Bits 'n Bobs

## Homemade Mayonnaise

2 tablespoons lemon juice
½ teaspoon Dijon mustard
1 whole egg
⅛ teaspoon paprika or 1 dash cayenne pepper (optional)
1 cup oil (macadamia nut oil or avocado oil preferred; the blade can turn olive oil very bitter)

Place the lemon juice, mustard, salt, and egg in a blender—also the paprika or cayenne, if desired. Blend at a high speed until the mixture starts to thicken, then slowly pour in the oil in a steady stream. You'll hear the pitch of your blender change as the mixture thickens, about 2 minutes. Scrape into a glass jar and refrigerate for 7–10 days.

## Baked Apples or Pears

6 apples or pears, cored and sliced
1 heaping teaspoon cinnamon
½ teaspoon cardamom
¼ teaspoon chili flakes (optional)
1 cup water
3 tablespoons butter

Preheat the oven to 350°F.

In an ovenproof dish place the sliced apples and pears. Pour the cinnamon, cardamom, chili flakes (if using), and water over the top. Add the butter.

Cover the baking dish and bake for 30 minutes.

Serve with coconut milk, chopped nuts, or cashew cream.

## Cashew Cream (sweet or savory)

2 cups raw cashews

1 cup cold water, plus more as needed

*Savory:*

1 teaspoon salt

2 tablespoons lemon juice

2 garlic cloves, crushed

1 teaspoon of chopped fresh herbs like chives, thyme, cilantro, mint, oregano, rosemary, basil

*Sweet:*

1 tablespoon maple syrup, coconut sugar, honey, or 1 pitted date

Cover the nuts with water and soak overnight. Drain nuts and put all the ingredients in a blender—add salt, lemon juice, fresh herbs, and garlic for a savory cream; for more of a sweet flavor, add maple syrup, coconut sugar, honey, or 1 pitted date.

Puree until thick and creamy. If too thick, gradually add water, starting with ⅓ cup, to thin it until desired consistency is achieved.

Variations: Substitiute with other nuts such as almonds, pecans, pistachios, or hazelnuts.

## Baba Ghanoush

3 tablespoons extra-virgin olive oil, divided

2 eggplants

Juice of 1 large lemon

⅓ cup tahini

2 garlic cloves, minced

Sea salt and freshly ground pepper, to taste

Preheat oven to 375°F. Rub 1 tablespoon olive oil over each eggplant and place on baking sheet, pricking holes in the skin with a fork. Roast for 30–40 minutes, turning occasionally, or until soft.

Remove from oven and allow to cool. Put the whole eggplants in a food processor; process for 5 minutes and then add lemon, tahini, and garlic. Process until creamy. Transfer to a bowl, season with salt and pepper, and slowly add the remaining 1 tablespoon of olive oil. Drizzle a bit on top of the Baba Ghanoush.

Yummy served with vegetables as a dip.

# Eggs

## Crust-less Quiche

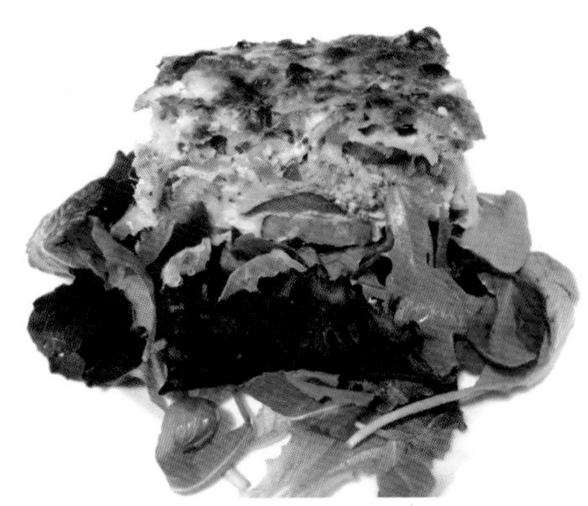

1 head cauliflower
6 eggs, beaten
Salt and pepper, to taste
1 teaspoon smoked paprika
1 tablespoon thyme, oregano, rosemary, or basil
1 tablespoon nutritional yeast (dairy-free)
¼ cup crumbled feta or Parmesan (optional)

Preheat oven to 350°F. Cut the cauliflower into small florets and spread in an ovenproof dish.

In a bowl whisk together eggs, salt and pepper to taste, paprika, and herbs.

Pour over the cauliflower and bake in the oven for 15 minutes.

Remove from the oven and sprinkle nutritional yeast, and feta or Parmesan cheese (if using) over the top.

Bake for another 5 minutes or until the cheese has melted.

# Coconut Egg Curry

1 cup grated coconut (sold frozen, thaw before cooking)
4 tablespoons coconut oil
¼ teaspoon cumin seeds
6 medium-sized pink shallots, sliced
¼-inch piece of fresh ginger, finely chopped
1 Thai chili (optional)
5 curry leaves
2 teaspoons coriander powder
1 teaspoon fennel powder
½ teaspoon garam masala powder
¼ teaspoon turmeric powder
1 tomato, diced
4 eggs
2 cups water
Salt, to taste

To make the coconut sauce:

Fry the grated coconut on medium heat until it turns golden. Once it cools down, grind this in a blender or food processor to make a fine powder. Add 1 cup of water to this powder and grind it for a couple of minutes to make a smooth paste. Set this aside.

In a pan, heat the coconut oil and sauté the cumin seeds. Once the seeds become fragrant, add the shallots, ginger, Thai chili, and curry leaves. When the shallots become translucent add the coriander, fennel, garam masala, and turmeric powder and mix well. Add the tomato and let it cook for a minute. To this mixture, add the coconut sauce. Add another cup of water, and salt to taste, and bring it to a boil. Mix it thoroughly. Now, one at a time, crack the eggs and drop them into different areas of the pan without much overlap. Do not stir. Keeping it covered, cook on a low flame for about 10 minutes. Stir gently and cook it for another 2 minutes. Remove from heat, stir and serve over white rice.

*(recipe by Aiswarya Palanisamy)*

# Baked Eggs in Tomato Sauce

⅓ cup of olive oil
2 onions chopped
3 garlic cloves minced
1 teaspoon dried oregano
1 teaspoon of cumin seeds
1 teaspoon of smoked paprika
1 teaspoon of chili flakes or
  ½ teaspoon of fresh chili, seeds removed and chopped
1 teaspoon of salt
½ teaspoon of pepper
2 pounds of ripe tomatoes, chopped,
  or one 28-ounce can of peeled tomatoes
4–6 eggs
1 bunch of Italian parsley chopped

In a Dutch oven sauté the onion, garlic, oregano, cumin seeds, smoked paprika, and chili flakes, until the onions are translucent.

Add the tomatoes, salt, and pepper and simmer for 45 minutes. If the sauce is too thick add ½–1 cup of water.

Remove from the heat and cool. Once cooled blend all the ingredients in a blender or food processor until smooth.

The sauce can be kept in a jar in the fridge for up to 1 week or frozen.

To cook the eggs:

Pour the sauce into a skillet and heat until bubbling, turn down the heat to medium, and with the back of a spoon make wells in the sauce. Crack the eggs into the wells, cover with a lid and cook for 5 minutes.

Scoop the tomato sauce and eggs into bowls and sprinkle with parsley.

# Egg Muffins

6 eggs

¼ pound cooked ground meat or sausage, or smoked salmon, or cooked turkey bacon, or shrimp

1 red pepper, finely chopped (or zucchini, spinach, mushrooms—in fact, any vegetables will work)

Salt and pepper to taste

Preheat oven to 350°F.

Generously grease 6 muffin tins with butter or coconut oil. Or for easier removal, line with paper baking cups. (They help the muffins hold their shape.)

In a bowl beat the eggs. Add meat, red pepper, and seasoning.

Spoon into muffin tins. Bake 18–20 minutes or until a knife stuck into the muffin comes out clean.

# Entrées

## Crab with Avocado and Ginger

Arugula
1 tablespoon olive oil
1 cup cooked crab meat
2 tablespoons pickled ginger
Zest and juice of 1 lemon
1 avocado, stoned and peeled, sliced

Dress the arugula with olive oil.

Mix together crab, ginger, lemon zest, and lemon juice.

Put the arugula in the center of the plate, avocado slices to the side, and top with crab.

## Ceviche

Juice of 2 lemons
Juice of 1 lime
1 small onion, finely chopped
1–2 fresh chilies, seeded and finely chopped
Salt and pepper, to taste
6 ounces salmon
6 ounces halibut or sea bass
6 ounces cod
6 ounces large shrimp
6 ounces scallops
½ avocado, stoned and cubed
2 tomatoes, skinned, seeded, and chopped
½ cup olive oil
½ cup roughly chopped coriander leaves

Mix the juice of the lemons and lime (save 1 tablespoon) with onion and chilies; add salt and pepper to taste.

Remove any skin, shells, or bones from the fish and cut into small cubes; cut shrimp in half.

Place the citrus marinade, fish, and shellfish in a sealable plastic bag—make sure the marinade coats all the fish. Place in the fridge for at least 5 hours. Turn the bag occasionally.

Drain the fish and shellfish and combine with the cubed avocado, tomatoes, olive oil, reserved tablespoon lemon/lime juice, and coriander. Add salt and pepper to taste.

# Cioppino

¼ cup olive oil
4 garlic cloves finely chopped
1 medium onion chopped
3 large shallots chopped
1 bay leaf
1 teaspoon dried thyme or 1 tablespoon fresh chopped
1 teaspoon dried red pepper flakes
1 teaspoon dried oregano or 1 tablespoon fresh chopped
2 teaspoons salt
1 teaspoon ground pepper
1 zested lemon and juice from the lemon
2 cups wine (red or white, depending on your preference)
5 cups chicken or fish stock
2 cans (14.5 ounces each) diced tomatoes in juice
1 pound clams scrubbed
1 pound of mussels scrubbed
1 ½ pounds large shrimp in the shell
1 ½ pounds assorted fish (halibut, cod, salmon) cut into bite-size chunks
2–4 cracked crab claws
1 ½ pounds of scallops
1 bunch of Italian parsley, roughly chopped

In a large pot or Dutch oven add the olive oil, onion, garlic, bay leaf, shallots, thyme, oregano, pepper flakes, salt, and pepper. Sauté on medium until onions are translucent.

Add lemon, lemon zest, wine, stock, and 2 cans of tomatoes and juice. Simmer for 1 hour. You may need to add additional stock or wine if the sauce gets too thick.

Add the clams and mussels to the stew; they should open within 5-10 minutes. Using tongs or a slotted spoon remove the open clams and mussels to a bowl and discard any that haven't opened.

Add the fish, shrimp, and scallops to the stew, simmer covered until just cooked through, about 5 minutes. Don't overcook.

Discard the bay leaf, and return the clams and mussels back to the pot. Gently stir in the parsley. Taste for more seasoning.

Note: for quicker Cioppino you can buy bottled Coppino sauces—to these add wine, herbs, and garlic—bring to a boil, then turn down to simmer and add any combination of fish and shellfish. Whole Foods sometimes sells fish for Cioppino, already cut up.

## Roasted Salmon or Red Snapper with Salsa

4 salmon or red snapper fillets (8 ounces each)
4 teaspoons olive oil, divided
1 tablespoon fresh lime juice
1 tablespoon cilantro, freshly chopped
Salt and pepper, to taste

Preheat oven to 400°F. Brush 1 teaspoon olive oil on a baking sheet and place fish skin-side down. Combine remaining olive oil, lime juice, and cilantro and brush on each fillet. Sprinkle with salt and pepper to taste.

Allow to sit for 15 minutes, then bake for 20 minutes, until just cooked. Garnish with salsa.

## Salsa

2 large tomatoes, diced
2 scallions, chopped
1 tablespoon cilantro, chopped
1 clove garlic, chopped
1 tablespoon olive oil
2 teaspoons fresh lime juice

Combine all ingredients in a bowl.

## Tea-poached Salmon with Herby Pesto

Coarse salt and freshly ground pepper, to taste
½ ounce loose tea, about 2 tablespoons (I like Lapson Souchon)
4 salmon fillets (4 ounces each), skinned (preferably wild)

Place salmon in a baking dish and sprinkle tea on top. Let stand 15 minutes at room temperature.

Bring 6 cups water to a boil. Generously salt water and return to a boil. Remove from heat and let cool to 160°F. (If water is too hot, fish will overcook.) Immediately pour enough hot water over fish to cover by 1 inch. Let stand 10 minutes for rare, or 12–13 minutes for medium rare. If water temperature gets below 140°F, add a little more hot water.

Using a slotted spoon, transfer fish to a paper towel–lined plate and pat dry. Spoon Herby Pesto (recipe below) over the fish and serve.

## Herby Pesto

1 cup parsley
¼ cup cilantro leaves
¼ cup basil leaves
¼ cup mint leaves
½ teaspoon ground cumin
½ teaspoon smoked paprika
2 cloves garlic minced
½ cup olive oil
Zest and juice of 1 lemon
¼ teaspoon of salt

Combine all the ingredients in a food processor.

# Salmon Cakes

1 pound skinned and boned fresh salmon
¼ cup finely chopped green onion (scallions)
¼ cup seeded and finely chopped red pepper
1 tablespoon crushed garlic
1 tablespoon finely chopped fresh oregano
1 tablespoon finely chopped fresh cilantro
1 tablespoon Dijon mustard
1 tablespoon capers
2 teaspoons salt
Zest and juice of 1 lemon
½ teaspoon freshly ground black pepper
¼ cup rice bran oil, grapeseed oil, avocado oil, or coconut oil

Combine all the ingredients in a food processor except the oil. Pulse until the mixture clumps together.

Form into cakes—makes about 6—and chill for 1 hour.

To bake in skillet:

Add oil to skillet and heat. Add the fish cakes and cook for 3 minutes; flip over for another 3 minutes. Serve with lemon dill sauce with a green salad.

To bake in oven:

Preheat the oven to 450°F. Grease a baking pan with olive oil and place in the hot oven. Remove the baking pan from the oven and place the salmon cakes on it—they should sizzle! Bake for 3 minutes on each side until golden brown. Serve with wasabi-ginger tartar sauce or lemon dill sauce with a green salad.

# Halibut Parcels with Chives

1 tablespoon olive oil
Zest and juice of 1 lemon
Salt and pepper, to taste
1 pound halibut
1 bunch chives, snipped

Preheat the oven to 350°F.

Mix oil, lemon juice and zest, salt, and pepper.

Portion the halibut, about ¼–½ pound per person.

Cut parchment paper for each portion, long enough to roll up.

Lay a halibut piece in the center of the parchment; pour 1 tablespoon of the lemon-oil mixture over the fish, and snip 1 teaspoon of chives over it.

Roll up the parchment like a parcel and place in the oven. Repeat with remaining portions.

Cook for 15 minutes. Place each parcel on a plate.

# Coconut Chicken

- 2 tablespoons olive oil or coconut oil
- 1 teaspoon finely chopped fresh ginger
- 1 teaspoon chili paste
- 1 teaspoon smoked paprika
- 1 heaped tablespoon garam masala or curry powder
- 1 onion, finely chopped
- 5 garlic cloves, chopped
- 8 chicken thighs
- 1 small potato, cut up into 1-inch cubes
- 1 (14-ounce) can coconut milk
- Zest and juice of 1 lime
- 1 bunch of Swiss chard, kale, or bok choy, washed and finely chopped
- Salt and pepper, to taste
- 1 bunch of mint, washed and finely chopped

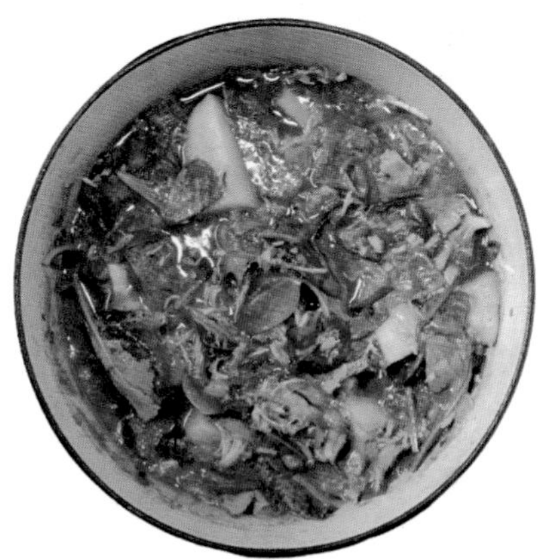

In a Dutch oven or large pot add 2 tablespoons of oil, ginger, chili paste, paprika, curry powder, and chopped onion. Sauté until translucent, then add garlic and cook for 1 minute.

Add chicken thighs, potatoes, and coconut milk and simmer for 20 minutes. If the broth gets too thick, dilute with ¼ cup of water.

Add chard, kale, or bok choy, and continue to cook for another 5 minutes. Add lime zest into coconut chicken, then add lime juice.

Serve garnished with chopped mint sprinkled on the top.

# Herby Chicken Patties

*makes about 8 patties*

1 ½ pounds ground white meat chicken

3 tablespoons chopped fresh sage

3 tablespoons chopped fresh oregano

Salt and pepper, to taste

2 green onions, chopped

2 tablespoons smoked paprika

4 garlic cloves, crushed or finely chopped

1 red pepper, finely chopped

1 knob ginger, about ½ inch, grated into the mixture or finely chopped (no need to peel)

2 tablespoons olive oil

Place all the ingredients in a food processor. Pulse 4–5 times.

Form into patties, brush with oil, and place on a hot grill—2–3 minutes on each side.

# Chicken Skewers with Artichoke and Lemon Pesto

Bamboo skewers soaked in water (stops from burning while grilling)
2 chicken breasts, cut into chunks and threaded onto skewers

*Marinade:*

1 tablespoon tamari sauce
1 tablespoon olive oil
3 garlic cloves, crushed
½ teaspoon chili flakes
Salt and pepper, to taste
Zest and juice of 1 lemon
1 cup of Lapson Souchon tea, cooled and strained
1 tablespoon maple syrup
Salt and pepper, to taste
1 tablespoon chopped fresh herbs (such as thyme/rosemary/mint/oregano)

Mix all the marinade ingredients together and pour over the skewered chicken. Leave for 4–8 hours.

Remove the skewers from the marinade and grill on a BBQ, or broil in the oven—about 8 minutes each side. Serve with Artichoke and Lemon Pesto (recipe follows).

# Artichoke Lemon Pesto

1 can artichoke hearts (in brine)
Juice and zest of 1 lemon
2 garlic cloves, crushed
¼ cup olive oil
Salt and pepper to taste

Drain the artichoke hearts and then process all the ingredients together in a blender or food processor. This is great as a dip for vegetables, or as a garnish for fish or chicken.

# Roasted Rosemary Chicken

1 whole chicken (organic, free range), giblets removed

3 bunches of rosemary

½ stick butter, softened

Salt and pepper, to taste

Preheat oven to 350°F.

Rinse and dry the chicken.

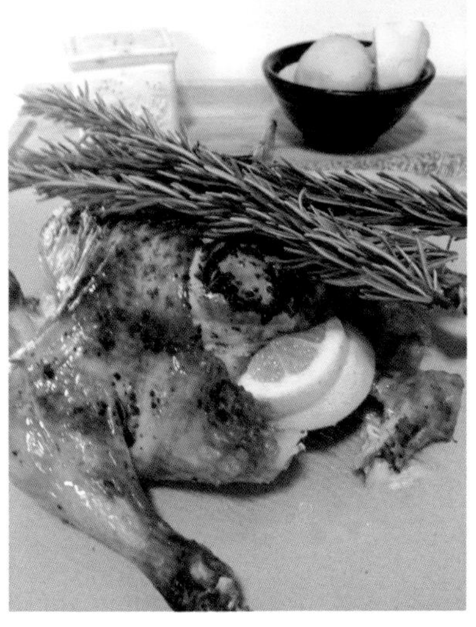

Roughly chop 2 bunches of the rosemary and mix into the butter. Rub the butter all over the chicken, including under the skin.

Place 2 stalks of rosemary in the chicken cavity.

Put the chicken in an ovenproof roasting dish and roast for 30 minutes; baste and roast for another 30 minutes—keep basting. Remove chicken from the oven and let stand for 15 minutes before serving.

Great for lunches.

# Roast Lamb

1 leg of lamb, deboned and butterfly-cut
4 cloves garlic, cut in slivers
1 bunch rosemary
1 teaspoon salt
½ teaspoon pepper
1 teaspoon dried oregano
1 lemon, zested and juiced

Poke holes in the lamb and insert garlic slivers and rosemary leaves.

Mix the salt, pepper, oregano, and lemon.

Grill on medium heat for about 20 minutes on each side.

Serve on a salad or with roasted vegetables.

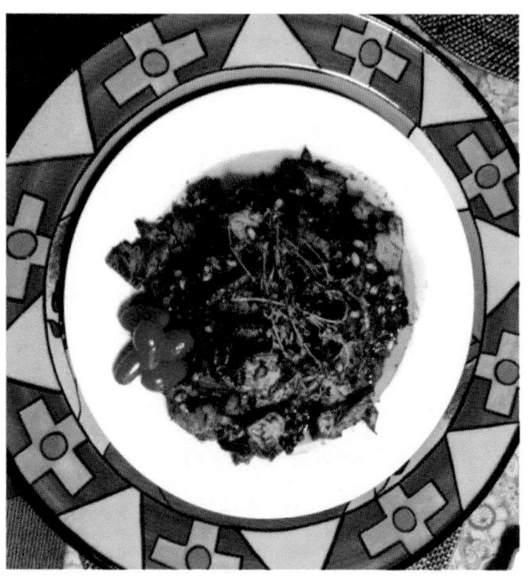

# Bobotie

Bobotie (buh-BOOT-ee) is a traditional South African Cape Malay dish of curried ground lamb with apricots, raisins, apples, and spices and a custard top. Don't be daunted by the list of ingredients; it's really easy and well worth it.

2 tablespoons olive oil
1 large onion, finely chopped
1–2 pounds ground lamb or beef, or a mixture of the two
4 garlic cloves, crushed
2 teaspoons turmeric
2 tablespoons masala or curry powder
2 teaspoons smoked paprika
2 teaspoons salt
½ teaspoon black pepper
1 heaping teaspoon cinnamon
1 teaspoon ground cumin
1 teaspoon powdered chili or flakes
½ cup golden raisins (or black)
½ cup of chopped dried apricots
Zest and juice of 1 lemon
2 tablespoons tomato paste
1 egg beaten
1 Granny Smith apple, peeled, cored, and chopped
3–4 bay or lemon leaves

Preheat the oven to 350°F.

Heat the oil in a large saucepan and sauté onions until golden.

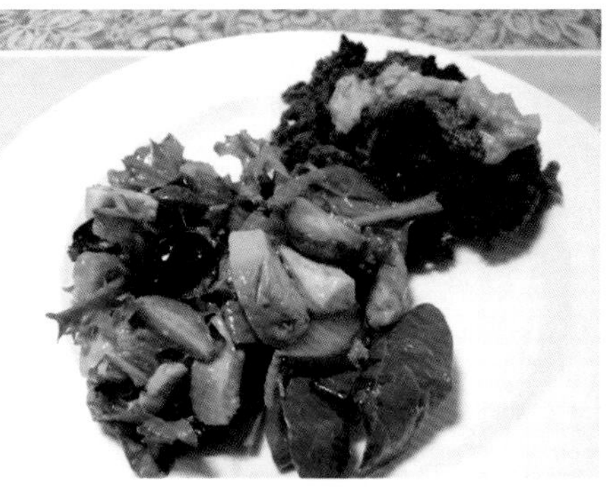

In a large mixing bowl, add all the ingredients except for the bay or lemon leaves: lamb, onion, garlic, spices, dried fruit, lemon juice and zest, tomato paste, egg, and apple. Mix well (I normally use my hands.)

Place mixture in a casserole dish; roll up the lemon or bay leaves and bury them in the bobotie.

Pat the top nice and flat. Cover with foil and bake for about 30 minutes, until the bobotie is firm and well cooked.

## Custard Topping

1 cup almond milk, coconut milk, or any nut milk
3 eggs
1 teaspoon salt

Mix together the milk, eggs, and salt, pour over the bobotie, and bake uncovered for about 15 minutes until set and lightly browned. Serve with Blatjang (chutney) and salad.

## Lamb Kofta

1 pound ground lamb
1 medium onion, finely chopped
Handful chopped parsley
1 teaspoon ground allspice
¼ teaspoon ground fenugreek
½ teaspoon ground red pepper
Salt, to taste
Oil for brushing
Lemon wedges
Tomatoes, sliced

Mix the meat, onion, parsley, allspice, fenugreek, pepper, and salt thoroughly in a large bowl.

Divide into 4–6 portions and, wetting your hands, form each into a sausage shape around a broad flat skewer. Brush each lightly with oil and grill for 10–15 minutes, turning the skewers from time to time. Serve the kofta with lemon wedges, olives, and sliced tomatoes.

# Asian Steak Salad

*Dressing:*

Zest and juice of 2 limes
1 tablespoon extra-virgin olive oil
1 tablespoon sesame oil
2 tablespoons water
2 tablespoons unseasoned rice vinegar

*Marinade:*

zest and juice of 1 lime
1 tablespoon freshly grated ginger
1 garlic clove, minced
2 scallions, thinly sliced (use some of the green)

*Salad:*

1 flank steak, large enough to equal 6 palm-sized portions
1 yellow bell pepper, cut into thin strips
1 small/medium head of Napa cabbage
⅓ cup fresh cilantro leaves
½ cup mint leaves, loosely packed
1 cup bean sprouts
2 tablespoons chopped pecans for garnish (optional)

*To make dressing:*

Whisk all the ingredients together in a small bowl; set aside.

*To make marinade:*

Whisk with all the ingredients in a shallow dish and cover steak with the marinade. Turn steak in the marinade and refrigerate for 1 hour. Let sit at room temperature for 30 minutes before grilling.

Heat a grill at medium-high. Cook about 5–7 minutes on each side, depending on thickness. Remove from grill when done to your preference. Cool for 5 minutes and slice thinly on the bias. In a salad bowl, combine the pepper, cabbage, cilantro, mint, and bean sprouts. Drizzle with dressing and toss well. Arrange veggies and steak on serving plates and garnish with some chopped pecans, if desired.

# Stir-fried Beef and Broccoli

2 tablespoons extra-virgin olive oil, divided
1–2 teaspoons finely minced fresh ginger
3 scallions, chopped (include some green)
2 garlic cloves, minced
1 pound flank steak, sliced across grain into thin strips
2 ½ cups broccoli florets
2 cups sliced mushrooms
1 medium yellow or red pepper
¾ cup beef broth
1 tablespoon arrowroot or tapioca
1 tablespoon dry white wine
2 tablespoons tamari soy sauce
Sea salt and freshly ground black pepper, to taste

In a wok, heat 1 tablespoon oil over medium-high heat. Add ginger and scallions, stir-frying for 1–2 minutes. Then add garlic and flank steak strips, stir-frying for 2 more minutes.

Remove from pan and set aside. Heat the remaining 1 tablespoon of oil in the wok over medium-high heat.

Add broccoli, mushrooms, and pepper. Quickly stir-fry for 1–2 minutes, then add beef broth.

Bring to a boil, cover, and reduce heat to a simmer until veggies are just tender (but not too soft), about 3–5 minutes. Return beef to pan. While veggies are cooking, mix arrowroot, wine, and soy sauce in a small bowl. Stir into wok and cook until thickened and heated through.

Add salt and pepper as needed.

# Burgers

1 ½ pounds of ground beef, buffalo, turkey, chicken, lamb, or pork, or a combination
1 onion, finely chopped
Salt and pepper to taste
*Optional:* 1 teaspoon smoked paprika; 1 teaspoon dried oregano, thyme, or rosemary
1 tablespoon oil

Into the ground meat, thoroughly mix the onion, herbs, and spices and form the meat into burgers.

Coat with oil to prevent sticking to a grill or hot pan. Serve with squash fries and green salad.

# Chili

1 onion, chopped
1 teaspoon of chili powder, or fresh chilies, seeds removed and finely chopped (start with less and slowly add more to accommodate your taste—it's always easier to add heat than try to remove it)
2 tablespoons olive oil
4 garlic cloves, crushed
1 teaspoon smoked paprika
2 tablespoons of ground cumin
2 pounds of ground beef, or combination of beef, turkey, pork, or lamb
1 (28-ounce) can of crushed tomatoes
1 teaspoon liquid smoke, or ½ cup steeped Lapson Souchon tea for a smoky flavor
2 cans kidney beans, drained
½ cup dark chocolate chips
2 tablespoons tomato paste
Salt and pepper, to taste

Sauté the onions and chopped chili (if using) in olive oil, until translucent; add ½ the garlic; add spices and continue to stir and cook for another 1–2 minutes.

Add the ground meat and canned tomatoes. You may need to break up the meat and tomatoes.

Add the liquid smoke or Lapson Souchon tea and canned beans.

Simmer for 30 minutes. Taste for more spices or heat—this is when to add more chili powder or chopped chilies as needed.

Add chocolate chips and continue to cook for another 10 minutes.

Add 2 tablespoons of tomato paste (this will thicken your chili, you may need to add more liquid—tea, water, or stock) and the other ½ of the garlic. Continue to cook for another 5 minutes. Adjust the seasoning, salt, and pepper to taste as needed.

Serve with cashew cream (page 228) and a green salad.

# Pork Satay

1 onion, finely chopped
1 knob of ginger, crushed or finely chopped
3 garlic cloves, pressed
1 tablespoon Chinese five-spice powder
4 tablespoons tamari or coconut aminos
1 tablespoon honey
6 tablespoons of coconut oil or olive oil
2 stalks lemongrass, finely sliced
1 pork tenderloin (2 pounds), cubed
Wooden or bamboo skewers (soaked) or metal skewers

Blend all the ingredients except pork (and skewers) to make a smooth marinade. Pour the marinade and coat the pork, and refrigerate for at least 2 hours.

Thread the meat onto the skewers and grill for 15–20 minutes. Turn them once or twice.

Serve with sriracha or any hot spicy sauce.

# Rice

## Slow Cooker Rice Porridge (Congee)

Also known as *jook*, congee turns up in Chinese households morning, noon, and night. This thick rendition is made heartier with the addition of chicken.

This very basic congee recipe is easy to customize by simply adding in your favorite chopped vegetables or meat a few minutes before serving. You can either use leftover meat that's cooked, or cook it in the congee for at least 15 minutes before serving. Be sure to use your favorite broth for this recipe—it brings most of the flavor to this dish.

2 cups uncooked rice (jasmine or brown rice)
4 cups water
4 cups broth
1 teaspoon salt
*Garnish:* chopped scallions and chopped cilantro,
sriracha or any other hot sauce

Rinse the rice well to clean it off. Combine the rice, water, broth, and salt in a slow cooker. Cook on low for 10–12 hours or until the rice has fallen apart and is soft in the broth. Ladle into bowls and garnish as you wish.

# Rice Pilaf

1 cup canned coconut milk—original, not low-fat or light
5 saffron threads, crushed into 1 tablespoon of warm water for 5 minutes
½ teaspoon ground cinnamon
¼ teaspoon black pepper
¼ teaspoon ground cloves
½ teaspoon cumin
2 curry leaves
Small piece of ginger (½ inch), finely chopped
Salt
4 tablespoons butter or ghee
1 ½ cups white jasmine or basmati rice (uncooked)
2 cups water

To the coconut milk add saffron, cinnamon, pepper, and cloves.

Heat the butter or ghee in a large pan or pot and stir in the cumin, curry leaves, and ginger. Add the rice and cook until it starts to turn brown, about 3–4 minutes.

Add the water, and bring to a boil, then simmer uncovered until virtually all the water is absorbed. Pour over the coconut milk/spice mixture.

Cover the top of the pot with foil and then the lid—turn the heat to very low and let simmer for 20 minutes.

# Malabar Rice

Malabar, India, is the home of cardamom and pepper, and this rice is a perfect accompaniment to chicken or lamb.

2 cups jasmine, basmati, or brown rice (uncooked)
3 cups water
2 tablespoons of ghee or oil
1 large onion finely chopped
8 green cardamom pods
2 cinnamon sticks, each broken into 3 pieces
8 cloves
1 teaspoon cumin seeds
12 black peppercorns
2 teaspoons salt

Cover the rice with the water for at least 30 minutes.

Heat the oil/ghee in a pan or a pot and sauté the onion until golden or translucent.

Bruise the cardamom pods (I use my garlic press; you can whack them with back of a heavy-handled knife).

Add cardamom, cinnamon, cloves, cumin, peppercorns, and salt to the onions and gently sauté for 2 minutes.

Drain the rice; reserve the water and add the rice to onions and herbs in the pan or pot and sauté for 3 minutes, and add the water.

Stir and bring to a boil, then reduce the heat to low. Cover the pan or pot and simmer for 20 minutes until all the water is absorbed.

Turn off the heat, replace the lid, and allow the rice to steam for another 10 minutes.

When ready to serve, turn out the rice onto a warmed platter; fluff with a wooden fork before serving.

# Vegetables

## Basic Recipe for Quick Steamed Greens

Choose any of the following: beet greens, bok choy, collard greens, dandelion greens, endive, kale, mustard greens, spinach, or Swiss chard. Servings will depend on the amount of greens used.

For greens with tough stems, tear or cut leaves away from the stem before washing. Wash carefully (fill sink with cold water, submerge greens, and rinse well). Chop into bite-size pieces.

Steam tender leaves for about 2–5 minutes, and tougher greens (kale, collards) for 5–10 minutes.

While greens are steaming, sauté 2–3 chopped cloves garlic in 1 tablespoon olive oil.

Toss steamed greens with olive oil and garlic.

Serve with a squeeze of fresh lemon, if desired.

For a different flavor:

- Add the zest and juice of 1 lemon into a bowl; add crushed garlic, oil, salt, pepper, and smoked paprika or chili.
- Add a sprinkle of cumin just before serving.
- Add 1 tablespoon of balsamic vinegar.
- Add 1 tablespoon of pesto.
- Add 1 teaspoon of garam masala mixed with 1 tablespoon of ghee.

## Red Cabbage with Apple and Cranberries

1 head red cabbage
3 tablespoons olive oil
1 teaspoon crushed garlic
1 bunch green onions, finely chopped
½ cup applesauce (unsweetened)
½ cup dried cranberries
1 tablespoon apple cider vinegar
Salt and pepper, to taste

Remove the outer leaves of the cabbage and cut the cabbage in half. Remove the center core. Slice the cabbage into ½-inch strips.

Heat the oil in a sauté pan; add the garlic, green onions, and cabbage. Sauté for 3 minutes; add the rest of the ingredients.

Sauté for another 5 minutes and serve.

## Brussels Sprouts

5 garlic cloves, crushed, divided
3 tablespoons olive oil, divided
1 tablespoon coconut aminos
Salt and pepper, to taste
½ teaspoon chili flakes
Zest and juice of 1 lemon
Juice of ½ orange
1 bag fresh brussels sprouts
Crisped bacon (optional)

Mix together 1 crushed garlic clove, 1 tablespoon olive oil, coconut aminos, salt, pepper, chili flakes, zest and juice of lemon, and juice of ½ orange and put aside.

Finely shred the brussels sprouts—the easiest way is to slice through the whole sprout, starting at the stem.

Heat the remaining oil in a sauté pan. Add the remaining garlic and cook for 1 minute; add the brussels sprouts. Stir-fry for about 3 minutes.

Remove from the pan and add the vinaigrette. Add crisped bacon, if desired.

## Roasted Garlic Broccoli

¼ cup avocado oil
½ teaspoon salt
¼ teaspoon pepper
5 garlic gloves minced
3–4 heads of broccoli cut into florets

Preheat oven to 450°F.

Combine oil, salt, pepper, and garlic in a large mixing bowl. Add the broccoli florets and thoroughly coat with the garlic mixture. Roast for 25 minutes.

## Rosemary Roasted Sweet Potatoes

¼ cup avocado oil
1 bunch fresh rosemary chopped (keep 1 teaspoon aside)
½ teaspoon salt
½ teaspoon pepper

Preheat the oven to 450°F.

Wash and dry the sweet potatoes (keep the peels on so you can get all those phytonutrients!) and then chop into 1-inch chunks.

Coat with oil, and mix in the rosemary.

Roast for 40 minutes, stirring halfway, or until the sweet potatoes are soft. Add salt, pepper, and 1 teaspoon of rosemary; mix thoroughly, being careful not to smash the potatoes.

## Mock Mashed Potatoes

1 head of cauliflower cut into florets
2 cups of chicken or beef stock
1 tablespoon of olive oil
Salt and pepper to taste

Simmer the cauliflower florets and stock in a large pot. After about 25 minutes, when the cauliflower is soft, mash the cauliflower and the remaining stock. Add salt and pepper to taste and, finally, add the olive oil. Mix well.

# Roasted Vegetables

1 head cauliflower
2 tablespoons olive oil or avocado oil
1 tablespoon finely chopped fresh mint
Salt and pepper, to taste

*Spice options for roasted vegetables:*
1 tablespoon turmeric
1 tablespoon curry powder
2 tablespoons smoked paprika
1 teaspoon cumin
1 teaspoon garlic salt
1 teaspoon lemon pepper
1 tablespoon cocoa powder (goes well on cauliflower)

Preheat oven to 400°F. Put 1 baking sheet into the oven.

Cut the cauliflower into small florets—you may have to discard the stem part in the middle, or save to put in soups.

Add oil, mint, salt, pepper, and your choice of spice in a large mixing bowl. Add the cauliflower and coat completely. I use my hands—messy, but fun and effective.

Pour the cauliflower onto the hot baking sheet—it should sizzle. Bake for 20 minutes.

You may also roast 4–6 different vegetables at a time, using 2–3 baking trays.

Tray 1: ⅓ cauliflower; ⅓ zucchini: oil, salt, pepper, and different spice; ⅓ peppers: cut with oil, salt, pepper, and different spice

Tray 2: ⅓ sweet potatoes: oil and fresh rosemary; ⅓ fennel: lemon juice and zest of lemon; ⅓ eggplant: oil and cumin

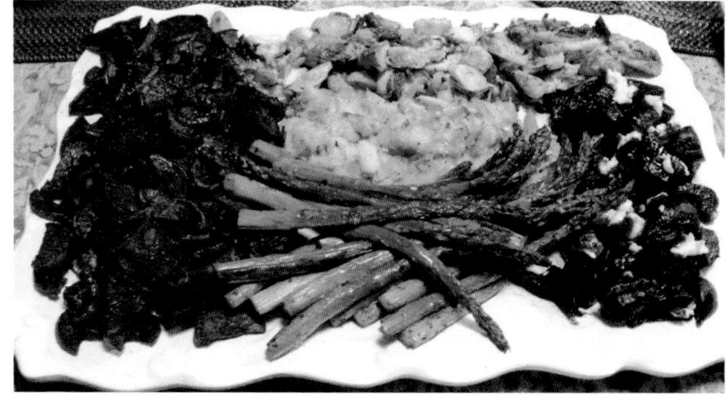

Bake for 20–30 minutes until the vegetables are cooked.

# Salads

Salads should never be boring if you add different and unusual things, and then dress well with different dressings. Make a few different dressings and alternate.

*Leafy greens*: mixed greens, arugula, romaine, butter lettuce, finely sliced Swiss chard, kale, bok choy, mustard greens, sprouts, and micro-greens.

*Other vegetables:* incorporate a few items from this list and try to rotate which vegetable you include: tomatoes, carrots, cucumber, celery, avocado, artichoke hearts (can), olives, cranberries, raisins, peppers, fruit, capers, onions, spring onions, garlic.

I love adding hot roasted vegetables to a salad—cauliflower, sweet potatoes, broccoli, beets, zucchini, eggplant, tomatoes, fennel, onions, garlic—and pouring a salad dressing on top.

*Nuts and seeds:* pine nuts, walnuts, almonds, cashews, pumpkin seeds, sunflower seeds.

*Herbs:* rosemary, basil, chives, mint.

*Protein:* eggs, chicken, turkey, smoked turkey, fish, shrimp, scallops, lamb, beef, chicken apple sausage.

# Salad Dressings

## Vinaigrette Dressing

1 teaspoon agave nectar
1 teaspoon of Dijon mustard
1/3–1/2 cup balsamic vinegar
2 cloves garlic, finely chopped or pressed
Salt and pepper, to taste
1/3 cup olive oil

Mix all the ingredients in a jar except the olive oil; shake well. Slowly add the olive oil and shake again.

Make a large bottle of the vinaigrette as a base. Add to salads or vegetables.

*Variations:*

- add more garlic for a delicious garlicky dressing
- add 1 tablespoon of olive tapenade
- add 1 tablespoon of pesto
- add 1 tablespoon of finely chopped rosemary or a mixture of herbs

## Tangy Tahini Dressing

½ cup cold-pressed extra virgin olive oil
½ cup tahini
2–3 tablespoons apple cider vinegar
Juice of ½ lemon
2 tablespoons water
1 teaspoon dried dill
1 teaspoon dried chives (optional)

Combine all the ingredients in a bottle with a tight lid and shake well. Will keep up to 2 weeks refrigerated.

## Smoky Lemon Tahini Dressing

*Tahini can vary in thickness, so you may need to add a little extra water to thin the dressing.*

*Makes 1 ½ cups*
2 garlic cloves, grated
½ cup tahini (sesame seed paste)
¼ cup fresh lemon juice
1 teaspoon sea salt
⅛ teaspoon smoked paprika

Purée garlic, tahini, lemon juice, salt, paprika, and ¾ cup water in a blender until smooth, adding water if needed to thin dressing.

## Citrus Vinaigrette

1 small shallot, finely chopped
¾ cup olive oil
¼ cup champagne vinegar
3 tablespoons fresh lemon juice
2 tablespoons fresh orange juice
¼ teaspoon finely grated lemon zest
Sea salt and freshly ground pepper, to taste

Combine first 6 ingredients in a small jar; season vinaigrette to taste with salt and pepper. Shake to blend.

# ACKNOWLEDGMENTS

If I had known how much work was involved in writing a book, I might have thought twice about undertaking the project. No, but seriously—it has been an incredibly rewarding experience, the most gratifying expression of my passion for writing, and the fulfillment of a lifelong dream. And it has also taken an army of people who have come together to make this dream a reality. There are far more people than I can mention individually here, but I hope that you know who you are and that you have my eternal gratitude.

To my agent, Jud Laghi, your commitment to this project from the beginning was unwavering and crucial. I thank you for the sage advice, insight, and wisdom you brought to every step of the process.

To my editor, Nicole Frail, and the entire team at Skyhorse Publishing, I thank you for facilitating the process and helping transform my rough ideas into the final print-ready version.

I would like to thank everyone at my clinic, the Institute for Health and Healing at California Pacific Medical Center in San Francisco, especially my director, Judith Tolson, for the unflagging support and encouragement. Sharon—your recipes are a critical part of this book, and I thank you for your culinary expertise and contribution!

I owe a debt of gratitude to many teachers, but I especially want to thank Dr. Andrew Weil for giving me a solid foundation in integrative medicine. I also want to thank my patients, who have been and continue to be my teachers.

My friends and family have been the biggest blessings in my life. I would like to thank my mom and dad for everything they have done for me. To my wife, Aiswarya, and my daughter, Alisha—thank you for inspiring me, loving me, and putting up with me patiently during all the long hours I spent on the computer. I am so lucky to have you both in my life. Everything I do and strive for—is for you.

# NOTES


## Introduction

1. Mark Hyman, *The Blood Sugar Solution* (New York: Little, Brown and Company, 2012).
2. "Allergy Facts and Figures," Asthma and Allergy Foundation of America, accessed March 20, 2015, http://www.aafa.org/display.cfm?id=9andsub=30.
3. A. Syed et al., "Food Allergy Diagnosis and Therapy: Where Are We Now?" *Immunotherapy* 5(9) (2013): 931–944.
4. Donna Jackson Nakazawa, *The Autoimmune Epidemic* (New York: Simon and Schuster, 2008), 24.
5. Jane Brody, "Celiac Disease, a Common, but Elusive, Diagnosis," *The New York Times,* September 29, 2014, http://well.blogs.nytimes.com/2014/09/29/celiac-disease-diagnosis-gluten/.
6. Martin Blaser, *Missing Microbes* (New York: Henry Holt and Company, 2014), 3.
7. Jason Kane, "Health Costs: How the US Compares with Other Countries," *PBS Newshour*, October 22, 2012, http://www.pbs.org/newshour/rundown/health-costs-how-the-us-compares-with-other-countries/.
8. Sarah Williams, "Gone Too Soon: What's Behind the High US Infant Mortality Rate," *Stanford Medicine* (2013), http://sm.stanford.edu/archive/stanmed/2013fall/article2.html.
9. J.A. Ricci et al., "Fatigue in the US Workforce: Prevalence and Implications for Lost Productive Work Time," *Journal of Occupational and Environmental Medicine* 49(1) (2007): 1.

## My Story

1. Rabindranath Tagore, *Fruit Gathering*, http://blog.gaiam.com/quotes/authors/rabindranath-tagore?page=1.

## Chapter 1

1. Gary Taubes, *Why We Get Fat and What to Do About It* (New York: Random House, 2011), 164.
2. Geoffrey Rose, "Strategy of Prevention: Lessons from Cardiovascular Disease," *British Medical Journal* 282(6279) (1981): 1851.
3. Loren Cordain et al. "Plant-animal subsistence ratios and macronutrient energy estimations in worldwide hunter-gatherer diets," *American Journal of Clinical Nutrition* 71(3) (2000): 682–692.

4. Paul Jaminet and Shou-Ching Jaminet, *Perfect Health Diet: Regain Health and Lose Weight by Eating the Way You Were Meant to Eat* (New York: Simon and Schuster, 2012), 10–11.
5. Weston Price, *Nutrition and Physical Degeneration* (Lemon Grove, CA: Price-Pottenger Nutrition Foundation, 1939).
6. Price, *Nutrition and Physical Degeneration.*
7. Dan Buettner, *The Blue Zones: Nine Lessons for Living Longer from the People Who've Lived the Longest* (Washington, DC: National Geographic Society, 2008).
8. Buettner, *The Blue Zones*, 118–119.
9. Buettner, *The Blue Zones*, 269.
10. Buettner, *The Blue Zones*,129.
11. Buettner, *The Blue Zones*, 223.
12. Buettner, *The Blue Zones*, 257.
13. Taubes, *Why We Get Fat and What to Do About It*, 169.
14. Taubes, *Why We Get Fat and What to Do About It*, 170–172.
15. Buettner, *The Blue Zones*, 117.

**Chapter 2**

1. Taubes, *Why We Get Fat and What to Do About It*, 138.
2. Fiona S. Atkinson, RD, et al., "International Tables of Glycemic Index and Glycemic Load Values: 2008," *Diabetes Care* 31(12) (2008): 2281–2283.
3. University of Sydney glycemic index group, www.glycemicindex.com.
4. M. Leeman et al., "Vinegar Dressing and Cold Storage of Potatoes Lowers Postprandial Glycaemic and Insulinaemic Responses in Healthy Subjects," *European Journal of Clinical Nutrition* 59(11) (2005): 1266.
5. C.J. Henry et al., "The Impact of the Addition of Toppings/Fillings on the Glycaemic Response to Commonly Consumed Carbohydrate Foods," *European Journal of Clinical Nutrition* 60(6) (2006): 763.
6. R.W. Simpson et al., "Macronutrients Have Different Metabolic Effects in Nondiabetics and Diabetics," *American Journal of Clinical Nutrition* 42(3) (1985): 449–453.
7. Henry et al., "The Impact of the Addition of Toppings/Fillings on the Glycaemic Response to Commonly Consumed Carbohydrate Foods," 763.
8. Michael Mosley and Mimi Spencer, *The Fast Diet* (New York: Simon and Schuster, 2013), 72.

9. S. Liu et al., "A Prospective Study of Dietary Glycemic Load, Carbohydrate Intake, and Risk of Coronary Heart Disease in US Women," *American Journal of Clinical Nutrition* 71(6) (2000): 1455–1461.

10. C.J. Tsai et al., "Dietary Carbohydrates and Glycaemic Load and the Incidence of Symptomatic Gall Stone Disease in Men," *Gut* 54(6) (2005): 823–828.

11. Henry et al., "The Impact of the Addition of Toppings/Fillings on the Glycaemic Response to Commonly Consumed Carbohydrate Foods," 763–769.

12. Ian Spreadbury, "Comparison with Ancestral Diets Suggests Dense Acellular Carbohydrates Promote an Inflammatory Microbiota, and May Be the Primary Dietary Cause of Leptin Resistance and Obesity," *Journal of Diabetes, Metabolic Syndrome and Obesity* 5 (2012): 175–189.

13. Taubes, *Why We Get Fat and What to Do About It*, 196.

14. Barry Sears with Bill Lawren, *The Zone: A Dietary Road Map* (New York: HarperCollins, 1995), 30–31.

15. Taubes, *Why We Get Fat and What to Do About It*, 10.

16. D.B. Boyd, "Insulin and Cancer," *Integrated Cancer Therapies* 2(4) (2003): 315–329.

17. J. L. Johnson et al., "Identifying prediabetes using fasting insulin levels," *Endocrine Practice* 16(1) (2010): 47–52.

18. Taubes, *Why We Get Fat and What to Do About It*, 19–32.

19. P. Nijeboer et al., "Non-Celiac Gluten Sensitivity: Is It in the Gluten or the Grain?" *Journal of Gastrointestinal and Liver Diseases* 22(4) (2013): 435–440.

20. J.A. Hawrelak et al., "Essential Oils in the Treatment of Intestinal Dysbiosis: A Preliminary In Vitro Study," *Alternative Medicine Review* 14(4) (2009): 380–384.

21. E.P. Halmos et al., "A Diet Low in Fodmaps Reduces Symptoms of Irritable Bowel Syndrome," *Gastroenterology* 146(1) (2014): 67–75.

22. J.R. Biesiekierski et al., "No Effects of Gluten in Patients with Self-Reported Non-Celiac Gluten Sensitivity After Dietary Reduction of Fermentable, Poorly Absorbed, Short-Chain Carbohydrates," *Gastroenterology* 145(2) (2013): 320–328.

23. C. Zioudrou et al., "Opioid Peptides Derived from Food Proteins: The Exorphins," *Journal of Biological Chemistry* 254(7) (1979): 2446–2449.

24. William Davis, *Wheat Belly* (New York: Rodale, 2011).

25. Jane Brody, "Celiac Disease, a Common, but Elusive, Diagnosis," *The New York Times,* September 29, 2014, http://well.blogs.nytimes.com/2014/09/29/celiac-disease-diagnosis-gluten/.
26. Blaser, *Missing Microbes,*175.
27. Blaser, *Missing Microbes,*175.
28. "Defending Traditional Grains," *Pathways 4 Health* (2012), http://pathways4health.org/2012/08/20/septemberoctober-2012-defending-wheat-restoring-wheat-2/#footnote_10_3384.
29. "Triticum Monococcum," Einkorn.com, October 1, 2012, http://www.einkorn.com/triticum-monococcum/.
30. Hyman, *The Blood Sugar Solution.*
31. David Perlmutter, *Grain Brain* (New York: Little, Brown and Company, 2013), 63.
32. H.C. van den Broeck et al., "Presence of Celiac Disease Epitopes in Modern and Old Hexaploid Wheat Varieties: Wheat Breeding May Have Contributed to Increased Prevalence of Celiac Disease," *Theoretical and Applied Genetics* 121(8) (2010): 1527–1539.
33. Hyman, *The Blood Sugar Solution.*
34. D. Pizzuti et al., "Lack of Intestinal Mucosal Toxicity of Triticum Monococcum in Celiac Disease Patients," *Scandinavian Journal of Gastroenterology* 41(11) (2006): 1305–1311.
35. D. Pizzuti et al., "Lack of Intestinal Mucosal Toxicity of Triticum Monococcum in Celiac Disease Patients," 1305–1311.
36. C.G. Rizzello et al., "Highly Efficient Gluten Degradation by Lactobacilli and Fungal Proteases during Food Processing: New Perspectives for Celiac Disease," *Applied and Environmental Microbiology* 73(14) (2007): 4499–4507.
37. Luigi Greco et al., "Safety for Patients with Celiac Disease of Baked Goods Made of Wheat Flour Hydrolyzed during Food Processing," *Clinical Gastroenterology and Hepatology* 9(1) (2011): 24–29.
38. Perlmutter, *Grain Brain,* 63.
39. Jaminet and Jaminet, *Perfect Health Diet: Regain Health and Lose Weight by Eating the Way You Were Meant to Eat,* 198–199.
40. M. Zwolińska-Wcisło et al., "Coeliac Disease and Other Autoimmunological Disorders Coexistence" [Article in Polish], *Przeglad Lekarski* 66(7) (2009): 370–372.
41. John McDougall, *The Starch Solution* (New York: Rodale, 2012), 8–10.

42. Abigail L. Mandel and Paul A.S. Breslin, "High Endogenous Salivary Amylase Activity Is Associated with Improved Glycemic Homeostasis Following Starch Ingestion in Adults," *Journal of Nutrition* 142(5) (2012), 853–858.
43. Elizabeth Brown, "Starchy Dangers in Human Evolution," *Science in the News,* Harvard Medical School, July 15, 2014, http://sitn.hms.harvard.edu/uncategorized/2014/starchy-dangers-in-human-evolution/.

**Chapter 3**

1. P.W. Siri-Tarino et al., "Meta-Analysis of Prospective Cohort Studies Evaluating the Association of Saturated Fat with Cardiovascular Disease," *American Journal of Clinical Nutrition* 91(3) (2010): 535–546.
2. Rajiv Chowdhury et al., "Association of Dietary, Circulating, and Supplement Fatty Acids with Coronary Risk: A Systematic Review and Meta-analysis," *Annals of Internal Medicine* 160 (2014): 398–406.
3. Ian A. Prior et al., "Cholesterol, Coconuts, and Diet on Polynesian Atolls: A Natural Experiment: The Pukapuka and Tokelau Island Studies," *American Journal of Clinical Nutrition* 34(8) (1981): 1552–1561.
4. A.G. Dulloo et al., "Twenty-four-hour Energy Expenditure and Urinary Catecholamines of Humans Consuming Low-to-Moderate Amounts of Medium-Chain Triglycerides: A Dose-Response Study in a Human Respiratory Chamber," *European Journal of Clinical Nutrition* 50(3) (1996): 152–158.
5. M.L. Assunção et al., "Effects of Dietary Coconut Oil on the Biochemical and Anthropometric Profiles of Women Presenting Abdominal Obesity," *Lipids* 44(7) (2009): 593–601.
6. B. Zhang et al., "The Relationships between Erythrocyte Membrane N-6 to N-3 Polyunsaturated Fatty Acids Ratio and Blood Lipids and C-Reactive Protein in Chinese Adults: An Observational Study," *Biomedical and Environmental Sciences* 24(3) (2011): 234–242.
7. M.A. Micallef et al., "An Inverse Relationship between Plasma N-3 Fatty Acids and C-Reactive Protein in Healthy Individuals," *European Journal of Clinical Nutrition* 63 (2009): 1154–1156.
8. Ramin Farzaneh-Far et al., "Inverse Association of Erythrocyte N-3 Fatty Acid Levels with Inflammatory Biomarkers in Patients with Stable Coronary Artery Disease: The Heart and Soul Study," *Atherosclerosis* 205 (2009): 538–543.

9. Catherine M. Alfano et al., "Fatigue, Inflammation, and ω-3 and ω-6 Fatty Acid Intake among Breast Cancer Survivors," *Journal of Clinical Oncology* 30(12) (2012): 1280–1287.

10. Sylvie S. Leung Yinko et al., "Fish Consumption and Acute Coronary Syndrome: A Meta-Analysis," *American Journal of Medicine* 127(9) (2014): 848–857.

11. W.S. Harris et al., "Comparison of the Effects of Fish and Fish-Oil Capsules on the N 3 Fatty Acid Content of Blood Cells and Plasma Phospholipids," *American Journal of Clinical Nutrition* 86(6) (2007): 1621–1625.

12. Kimberly M. Carlson "Committed Carbon Emissions, Deforestation, and Community Land Conversion from Oil Palm Plantation Expansion in West Kalimantan, Indonesia," *Proceedings of the National Academy of Sciences* 109(19) (2012): 7559–7564.

13. Rebecca Smith, "Full Fat Milk and Cheese Reduce the Risk of Diabetes: Study," *The Telegraph,* September 16, 2014, http://www.telegraph.co.uk/health/healthnews/11096655/Full-fat-milk-and-cheese-reduce-the-risk-of-diabetes-study.html.

14. M.A. Pereira et al., "Dairy Consumption, Obesity and the Insulin Resistance Syndrome in Young Adults: The Cardia Study," *JAMA: The Journal of the American Medical Association* 287 (2002): 2081–2089.

15. Hyon K. Choi et al., "Dairy Consumption and Risk of Type 2 Diabetes Mellitus in Men: A Prospective Study," *Archives of Internal Medicine* 165 (2005): 997–1003.

16. D. Mozaffarian et al., "Trans-Palmitoleic Acid, Metabolic Risk Factors, and New-Onset Diabetes in US Adults: A Cohort Study," *Annals of Internal Medicine* 153(12) (2010): 790–799.

17. J.E. Chavarro et al., "A Prospective Study of Dairy Foods Intake and Anovulatory Infertility," *Human Reproduction* 22(5) (2007): 1340–1347.

18. Catharine Paddock, "Reduced Fertility in Women Linked to Low Fat Dairy Food," *Medical News Today,* March 1, 2007, http://www.medicalnewstoday.com/articles/64192.php.

19. D.S. Weigle, "A High-Protein Diet Induces Sustained Reductions in Appetite, Ad Libitum Caloric Intake, and Body Weight Despite Compensatory Changes in Diurnal Plasma Leptin and Ghrelin Concentrations," *American Journal of Clinical Nutrition* 82(1) (2005): 41–48.

20. McDougall, *The Starch Solution*, 8.

21. McDougall, *The Starch Solution.*
22. L. Djoussé and J.M. Gaziano, "Dietary Cholesterol and Coronary Artery Disease: A Systematic Review," *Current Atherosclerosis Reports* 11(6) (2009): 418–422.
23. Thomas Remer, "Influence of Diet on Acid-Base Balance," *Seminars in Dialysis* 13(4) (2000): 221–226.
24. Thomas Remer et al., "Dietary Protein's and Dietary Acid Load's Influence on Bone Health," *Critical Reviews in Food Science and Nutrition* 54(9) (2014): 1140–1150.
25. U.S. Barzel and L.K. Massey, "Excess Dietary Protein Can Adversely Affect Bone," *Journal of Nutrition* 128(6) (1998): 1051–1053.
26. R.P. Heaney and D.K. Layman, "Amount and Type of Protein Influences Bone Health," *American Journal of Clinical Nutrition* 87(5) (2008): 1567S–1570S.
27. Renata Micha, et al., "Red and Processed Meat Consumption and Risk of Incident Coronary Heart Disease, Stroke, and Diabetes Mellitus: A Systematic Review and Meta-analysis," *Circulation* 121(21) (2010): 2271–2283.

**Chapter 4**

1. Sandi Busch, "What Green Lettuce Is the Most Nutritious?" http://healthyeating.sfgate.com/green-lettuce-nutritious-4316.html.
2. North Carolina Potato Association, "Consumer Information," http://www.ncagr.gov/markets/commodit/horticul/potatoes/facts.htm.
3. Nature's Sunshine, "What the Average American Eats in a Year," http://blog.naturessunshine.com/what-are-we-eating/.
4. "What Is the Special Nutritional Power Found in Fruits and Vegetables?" The World's Healthiest Foods. http://www.whfoods.com/genpage.php?tname=faqanddbid=4.
5. J. Kanner et al., "Betalains—A New Class of Dietary Cationized Antioxidants," *Journal of Agriculture and Food Chemistry* 49(11) (2001): 5178–5185.
6. "Cruciferous Vegetables and Cancer Prevention," National Cancer Institute, http://www.cancer.gov/cancertopics/causes-prevention/risk-factors/diet/cruciferous-vegetables-fact-sheet.
7. Jo Robinson, *Eating on the Wild Side: The Missing Link to Optimum Health* (New York: Little, Brown and Company, 2013).
8. Loren Cordain, *The Paleo Answer: 7 Days to Lose Weight, Feel Great, Stay Young* (Hoboken, NJ: John Wiley and Sons, 2012), 29.
9. Robinson, *Eating on the Wild Side, 216-217.*

10. Mohammad R. Vafa et al., "Effects of Apple Consumption on Lipid Profile of Hyperlipidemic and Overweight Men" *International Journal of Preventive Medicine* 2(2) (2011): 94–100.
11. H.M. Kang and M.E. Saltveit, "Antioxidant Capacity of Lettuce Leaf Tissue Increases after Wounding," *Journal of Agricultural and Food Chemistry* 50(26) (2002): 7536–7541.
12. "Carrots are the Food of the Week," The World's Healthiest Foods. http://www.whfoods.com/genpage.php?tname=foodspice&dbid=21.
13. Amanda Rose, "Phytic Acid – Soaking beans," January 20, 2010 http://www.phyticacid.org/soaking-beans/.
14. L. Wang et al., "Effect of a Moderate Fat Diet with and without Avocados on Lipoprotein Particle Number, Size and Subclasses in Overweight and Obese Adults: A Randomized, Controlled Trial," *Journal of the American Heart Association* 4(1) (2015).

**Chapter 5**

1. Shaun Marsh, "Doctors from Many Hospitals Prescribe Too Many Unnecessary Antibiotics: Study," Capital OTC, September 10, 2014, http://www.capitalotc.com/doctors-from-many-hospitals-prescribe-too-many-unnecessary-antibiotics-study/22080/.
2. Blaser, *Missing Microbes.*
3. Blaser, *Missing Microbes*, 79–82.
4. Blaser, *Missing Microbes*, 85.
5. Case Adams, *Probiotics: Protection Against Infection* (Wilmington, DE: Logical Books, 2012), 230–234.
6. Adams, *Probiotics: Protection Against Infection,* 230–231.
7. A. Chao et al., "Meat Consumption and Risk of Colorectal Cancer," *JAMA: The Journal of the American Medical Association* 293(2) (2005): 172–182.
8. Adams, *Probiotics: Protection Against Infection.*
9. Moises Velasquez-Manoff, *An Epidemic of Absence: A New Way of Understanding Allergies and Autoimmune Diseases* (New York: Simon and Schuster, 2012), 110.
10. Velasquez-Manoff, *An Epidemic of Absence*, 113.
11. Matt Ridley, "Dirtier Lives May Be Just the Medicine We Need," *The Wall Street Journal*, September 7, 2012, http://online.wsj.com/news/articles/SB10000872396390443686004577633400584241864.

12. Blaser, *Missing Microbes*, 138–139.
13. Adams, *Probiotics: Protection Against Infection,* 210–211.
14. Blaser, *Missing Microbes.*
15. R. Randal Bollinger et al., "Biofilms in the Large Bowel Suggest an Apparent Function of the Human Vermiform Appendix," *Journal of Theoretical Biology* 249(4) (2007): 826–831.
16. R. Satish Kumar et al., "Traditional Indian Fermented Foods: A Rich Source of Lactic Acid Bacteria," *International Journal of Food Sciences and Nutrition* 64(4) (2013):415-28.
17. A. A. Mohammadi et al., "The Effects of Probiotics on Mental Health and Hypothalamic-pituitary-adrenal Axis: A Randomized, Double-blind, Placebo-controlled Trial in Petrochemical Workers," *Nutritional Neuroscience* April 16, 2015 [Epub ahead of print].
18. M.R. Hilimire et al., "Fermented Foods, Neuroticism, and Social Anxiety: An Interaction Model," *Psychiatry Research* 228(2) (2015):203–8.
19. Adams, *Probiotics: Protection Against Infection,* 234–236.
20. Adams, *Probiotics: Protection Against Infection,* 236.
21. Günther Boehm and Bernd Stahl, "Oligosaccharides from Milk," *Journal of Nutrition* 137(3) (2007): 847S–849S.
22. Newswise, "New Low-Calorie Rice Could Help Cut Rising Obesity Rates, " source: American Chemical Society, March 23, 2015, http://www.newswise.com/articles/new-low-calorie-rice-could-help-cut-rising-obesity-rates.
23. Matthew Austin et al., "Fecal Microbiota Transplantation in the Treatment of *Clostridium Difficile* Infections," *American Journal of Medicine* 127(6) (2014): 479–483.
24. Austin et al., "Fecal Microbiota Transplantation in the Treatment of *Clostridium Difficile* Infections," 479–483.

**Chapter 7**

1. Michael Ristow, "Unraveling the Truth About Antioxidants: Mitohormesis Explains ROS-induced Health Benefits," *Nature Medicine* 20 (2014): 709–711.
2. H.J. Forman et al., "How Do Nutritional Antioxidants Really Work? Nucleophilic Tone and Para-Hormesis Versus Free Radical Scavenging In Vivo," *Free Radical Biology and Medicine* 66 (2014): 24–35.
3. Marc Birringer, "Hormetics: Dietary Triggers of an Adaptive Stress Response," *Pharmaceutical Research* 28(11) (2011): 2680–2694.

4. S.B. Lotito and B. Frei, "Consumption of Flavonoid-rich Foods and Increased Plasma Antioxidant Capacity in Humans: Cause, Consequence, or Epiphenomenon?" *Free Radical Biology and Medicine* 241(12) (2006): 1727–1746.
5. S. Czernichow et al., "Effects of Long-Term Antioxidant Supplementation and Association of Serum Antioxidant Concentrations with Risk of Metabolic Syndrome in Adults," *American Journal of Clinical Nutrition* 90(2) (2009): 329–335.
6. Bharat B. Aggarwal and Shishir Shishodia, "Suppression of the Nuclear Factor-κB Activation Pathway by Spice-derived Phytochemicals: Reasoning for Seasoning," *Annals of the New York Academy of Sciences* 1030 (2004): 434–441.
7. Shishir Shishodia et al., "Curcumin: Getting Back to the Roots," *Annals of the New York Academy of Sciences* 1056 (2005): 206–217.
8. V. Kuptniratsaikul et al., "Efficacy and Safety of Curcuma Domestica Extracts Compared with Ibuprofen in Patients with Knee Osteoarthritis: A Multicenter Study," *Clinical Interventions in Aging* 9 (2014): 451–458.
9. B. Chandran and A. Goel, "A Randomized, Pilot Study to Assess the Efficacy and Safety of Curcumin in Patients with Active Rheumatoid Arthritis," *Phytotherapy Research* 26(11) (2012): 1719–1725.
10. B. Lal et al., "Efficacy of Curcumin in the Management of Chronic Anterior Uveitis," *Phytotherapy Research* 13(4) (1999): 318–322.
11. R. Agarwal et al., "Detoxification and Antioxidant Effects of Curcumin in Rats Experimentally Exposed to Mercury," *Journal of Applied Toxicology* 30 (2010): 457–468.
12. Bharat Aggarwal with Debora Yost, *Healing Spices: How to Use 50 Everyday and Exotic Spices to Boost Health and Beat Disease* (New York: Sterling, 2011), 243.
13. W. Wongcharoen and A. Phrommintikul, "The Protective Role of Curcumin in Cardiovascular Diseases," *International Journal of Cardiology* 133(2) (2009): 145–151.
14. N. Akazawa et al., "Curcumin Ingestion and Exercise Training Improve Vascular Endothelial Function in Postmenopausal Women," *Nutritional Research* 32(10) (2012): 795–799.
15. P. Usharani et al., "Effect of NCB-02, Atorvastatin and Placebo on Endothelial Function, Oxidative Stress and Inflammatory Markers in Patients with Type 2 Diabetes Mellitus: A Randomized, Parallel-group, Placebo-controlled, 8-Week Study," *Drugs in R&D* 9(4) (2008): 243–250.

16. W. Wongcharoen et al., "Effects of Curcuminoids on Frequency of Acute Myocardial Infarction after Coronary Artery Bypass Grafting," *American Journal of Cardiology* 110(1) (2012): 40–44.
17. S. Mishra and K. Palanivelu, "The Effect of Curcumin (Turmeric) on Alzheimer's Disease: An Overview," *Annals of Indian Academy of Neurology* 11(1) (2008): 13–19.
18. R.B. Mythri and M.M. Bharath, "Curcumin: A Potential Neuroprotective Agent in Parkinson's Disease," *Current Pharmaceutical Design* 18(1) (2012): 91–99.
19. Xu Ying et al., "Curcumin Reverses the Effects of Chronic Stress on Behavior, the HPA Axis, BDNF Expression and Phosphorylation of CREB," *Brain Research* 1122(1) (2006): 56–64.
20. Mishra and Palanivelu, "The Effect of Curcumin (Turmeric) on Alzheimer's Disease: An Overview," 13–19.
21. Aggarwal with Yost, *Healing Spices*, 249.
22. Bharat B. Aggarwal et al., "Curcumin-Free Turmeric Exhibits Anti-Inflammatory and Anticancer Activities: Identification of Novel Components of Turmeric," *Molecular Nutrition and Food Research* 57(9) (2013): 1529–1542.
23. Mishra and Palanivelu, "The Effect of Curcumin (Turmeric) on Alzheimer's Disease: An Overview," 13–19.
24. Mishra and Palanivelu, "The Effect of Curcumin (Turmeric) on Alzheimer's Disease: An Overview," 13–19.
25. G. Shoba et al., "Influence of Piperine on the Pharmacokinetics of Curcumin in Animals and Human Volunteers," *Planta Medica* 64(4) (1998): 353–356.
26. P. Karna et al., "Benefits of Whole Ginger Extract in Prostate Cancer," *British Journal of Nutrition* 107(4) (2012): 473–484.
27. K.L. Wu et al., "Effects of Ginger on Gastric Emptying and Motility in Healthy Humans," *European Journal of Gastroenterology and Hepatology* 20(5) (2008): 436–440.
28. E. Ernst and M.H. Pittler, "Efficacy of Ginger for Nausea and Vomiting: A Systematic Review of Randomized Clinical Trials," *British Journal of Anaesthesia* 84(3) (2000): 367–371.
29. G. Paramdeep, "Efficacy and Tolerability of Ginger (Zingiber Officinale) in Patients of Osteoarthritis of Knee," *Indian Journal of Physiology and Pharmacology* 57(2) (2013): 177–183.
30. R.D. Altman and K.C. Marcussen, "Effects of a Ginger Extract on Knee Pain in Patients with Osteoarthritis," *Arthritis and Rheumatology* 44(11) (2001): 2531–2538.

31. C.D. Black et al., "Ginger (Zingiber Officinale) Reduces Muscle Pain Caused by Eccentric Exercise," *Journal of Pain* 11(9) (2010): 894–903.

32. Giti Ozgoli et al., "Comparison of Effects of Ginger, Mefenamic Acid, and Ibuprofen on Pain in Women with Primary Dysmenorrhea," *Journal of Alternative and Complementary Medicine* 15(2) (2009): 129–132.

33. J. Citronberg et al., "Effects of Ginger Supplementation on Cell-cycle Biomarkers in the Normal-appearing Colonic Mucosa of Patients at Increased Risk for Colorectal Cancer: Results from a Pilot, Randomized, and Controlled Trial," *Cancer Prevention Research* (Phila) 6(4) (2013): 271–281.

34. Karna et al., "Benefits of Whole Ginger Extract in Prostate Cancer," 473–484.

35. J. Rhode, "Ginger Inhibits Cell Growth and Modulates Angiogenic Factors in Ovarian Cancer Cells," *BMC Complementary and Alternative Medicine* 7 (2007): 44.

36. T. Arablou et al., "The Effect of Ginger Consumption on Glycemic Status, Lipid Profile and Some Inflammatory Markers in Patients with Type 2 Diabetes Mellitus," *International Journal of Food Sciences and Nutrition* 65(4) (2014): 515–520.

37. N. Khandouzi et al., "The Effects of Ginger on Fasting Blood Sugar, Hemoglobin A1c, Apolipoprotein B, Apolipoprotein A-I and Malondialdehyde in Type 2 Diabetic Patients," *Iran Journal of Pharmaceutical Research* 14(1) (2015): 131–140.

38. J.S. Chang et al., "Fresh Ginger (Zingiber Officinale) has Anti-viral Activity against Human Respiratory Syncytial Virus in Human Respiratory Tract Cell Lines," *Journal of Ethnopharmacology* 145(1) (2013): 146–151.

39. Ponmurugan Karuppiah and Shyamkumar Rajaram, "Antibacterial Effect of *Allium Sativum* Cloves and *Zingiber Officinale* Rhizomes against Multiple-drug Resistant Clinical Pathogens," *Asian Pacific Journal of Tropical Biomedicine* 2(8) (2012): 597–601.

40. Naritsara Saenghong et al., "*Zingiber Officinale* Improves Cognitive Function of the Middle-aged Healthy Woman," *Evidence-Based Complementary and Alternative Medicine* 2012 (2012): 383062.

41. P. Krüth et al., "Ginger-associated Overanticoagulation by Phenprocoumon," *Annals of Pharmacotherapy* 38(2) (2004): 257–260.

42. J.O. Ciocon et al., "Dietary Supplements in Primary Care: Botanicals Can Affect Surgical Outcomes and Follow-up," *Geriatrics* 59(9) (2004): 20–24.

43. B. Shan et al., "Antioxidant Capacity of 26 Spice Extracts and Characterization of Their Phenolic Constituents," *Journal of Agriculture and Food Chemistry* 53(20) (2005): 7749–7759.

44. S.A. Kouzi et al., "Natural Supplements for Improving Insulin Sensitivity and Glucose Uptake in Skeletal Muscle," *Frontiers in Bioscience* (Elite Ed) 7 (2015): 107–121.

45. R.W. Allen et al., "Cinnamon Use in Type 2 Diabetes: An Updated Systematic Review and Meta-analysis," *Annals of Family Medicine* 11(5) (2013): 452–459.

46. The World's Healthiest Foods, "Cinnamon," http://www.whfoods.com/genpage.php?tname=foodspiceanddbid=68.

47. P.V. Rao and S.H. Gan, "Cinnamon: A Multifaceted Medicinal Plant," *Evidence-based Complementary and Alternative Medicine: eCAM* 2014 (2014): 642942.

48. Rao and Gan, "Cinnamon: A Multifaceted Medicinal Plant," 642942.

49. J.G. Wang et al., "The Effect of Cinnamon Extract on Insulin Resistance Parameters in Polycystic Ovary Syndrome: A Pilot Study," *Fertility and Sterility* 88(1) (2007): 240–243.

50. J.M. Quale et al., "In Vitro Activity of Cinnamomum Zeylanicum against Azole Resistant and Sensitive Candida Species and a Pilot Study of Cinnamon for Oral Candidiasis," *American Journal of Chinese Medicine* 24(2) (1996): 103–109.

51. B. Ouattara et al., "Antibacterial Activity of Selected Fatty Acids and Essential Oils Against Six Meat Spoilage Organisms," *International Journal of Food Microbiology* 37(2–3) (1997): 155–162.

52. "High Daily Intakes of Cinnamon: Health Risk Cannot Be Ruled Out," BfR Health Assessment No. 044/2006, August 2006, www.bfr.bund.de/cm/349/high_daily_intakes_of_cinnamon_health_risk_cannot_be_ruled_out.pdf.

53. "Frequently Asked Questions about Coumarin in Cinnamon and Other Foods," The German Federal Institute for Risk Assessment, October 2006, http://www.bfr.bund.de/cm/349/frequently_asked_questions_about_coumarin_in_cinnamon_and_other_foods.pdf.

54. K.G. Samani and E. Farrokhi, "Effects of Cumin Extract on Oxldl, Paraoxanase 1 Activity, FBS, Total Cholesterol, Triglycerides, HDL-C, LDL-C, Apo A1, and Apo B in the Patients with Hypercholesterolemia," *International Journal of Health Sciences* (Qassim) 8(1) (2014): 39–43.

55. The World's Healthiest Foods, "Cumin Seeds," http://www.whfoods.com/genpage.php?tname=foodspiceanddbid=91.

56. K. Srinivasan, "Plant Foods in the Management of Diabetes Mellitus: Spices as Beneficial Antidiabetic Food Adjuncts," *International Journal of Food Sciences and Nutrition* 56(6) (2005): 399–414.

57. M. Saraswat et al., "Prevention of Non-enzymic Glycation of Proteins by Dietary Agents: Prospects for Alleviating Diabetic Complications," *British Journal of Nutrition* 101(11) (2009): 1714–1721.

58. Samani and Farrokhi, "Effects of Cumin Extract on Oxldl, Paraoxanase 1 Activity, FBS, Total Cholesterol, Triglycerides, HDL-C, LDL-C, Apo A1, and Apo B in the Patients with Hypercholesterolemia," 39–43.

59. Aggarwal with Yost, *Healing Spices*, 108.

60. S.S. Shirke et al., "Methanolic Extract of Cuminum Cyminum Inhibits Ovariectomy-induced Bone Loss in Rats," *Experimental Biology and Medicine* (Maywood) 233(11) (2008): 1403–1410.

61. N.S. Iacobellis et al., "Antibacterial Activity of Cuminum Cyminum L. and Carum Carvi L. Essential Oils," *Journal of Agriculture and Food Chemistry* 53(1) (2005): 57–61.

62. Aggarwal with Yost, *Healing Spices*, 47–48.

63. B.H. Ali and G. Blunden, "Pharmacological and Toxicological Properties of Nigella Sativa," *Phytotherapy Research* 17(4) (2003): 299–305.

64. H. Kaatabi et al., "Nigella Sativa Improves Glycemic Control and Ameliorates Oxidative Stress in Patients with Type 2 Diabetes Mellitus: Placebo Controlled Participant Blinded Clinical Trial," *PLoS ONE* 10(2) (2015): e0113486.

65. H. Fallah Huseini et al., "Blood Pressure Lowering Effect of Nigella Sativa L. Seed Oil in Healthy Volunteers: A Randomized, Double-blind, Placebo-controlled Clinical Trial," *Phytotherapy Research* 27(12) (2013): 1849–1853.

66. Kaatabi et al., "Nigella Sativa Improves Glycemic Control and Ameliorates Oxidative Stress in Patients with Type 2 Diabetes Mellitus," e0113486.

67. Ali M. Sabzghabaee et al., "Clinical Evaluation of Nigella Sativa Seeds for the Treatment of Hyperlipidemia: A Randomized, Placebo Controlled Clinical Trial," *Medical Archives* 66(3) (2012): 198–200.

68. R.M. Ibrahim et al., "A Randomised Controlled Trial on Hypolipidemic Effects of Nigella Sativa Seeds Powder in Menopausal Women," *Journal of Translational Medicine* 12 (2014): 82.

69. T.A. Gheita and S.A. Kenawy, "Effectiveness of Nigella Sativa Oil in the Management of Rheumatoid Arthritis Patients: A Placebo Controlled Study," *Phytotherapy Research* 26(8) (2012): 1246–1248.

70. H. Mahmoudvand et al., "Evaluation of Antifungal Activities of the Essential Oil and Various Extracts of Nigella Sativa and Its Main Component, Thymoquinone

against Pathogenic Dermatophyte Strains," *Journal de Mycologie Médicale* 24(4) (2014): e155–161.

71. M. Kolahdooz et al., "Effects of Nigella Sativa L. Seed Oil on Abnormal Semen Quality in Infertile Men: A Randomized, Double-blind, Placebo-controlled Clinical Trial," *Phytomedicine* 21(6) (2014): 901–905.
72. Ali and Blunden, "Pharmacological and Toxicological Properties of Nigella Sativa," 299–305.
73. M. Aqel and R. Shaheen, "Effects of the Volatile Oil of Nigella Sativa Seeds on the Uterine Smooth Muscle of Rat and Guinea Pig," *Journal of Ethnopharmacology* 52(1) (1996): 23–26.
74. S.I. Rizvi and N. Mishra, "Traditional Indian Medicines Used for the Management of Diabetes Mellitus," *Journal of Diabetes Research* 2013 (2013): 712092.
75. Aggarwal with Yost, *Healing Spices*, 119.
76. Nithya Neelakantan et al., "Effect of Fenugreek (Trigonella *Foenum-Graecum* L.) Intake on Glycemia: A Meta-analysis of Clinical Trials," *Nutrition Journal* 13 (2014): 7.
77. J.N. Losso et al., "Fenugreek Bread: A Treatment for Diabetes Mellitus," *Journal of Medicinal Food* 12(5) (2009): 1046–1049.
78. N. Kassaian et al., "Effect of Fenugreek Seeds on Blood Glucose and Lipid Profiles in Type 2 Diabetic Patients," *International Journal for Vitamin and Nutrition Research* 79(1) (2009): 34–39.
79. A. Gupta et al., "Effect of *Trigonella Foenum-Graecum* (Fenugreek) Seeds on Glycaemic Control and Insulin Resistance in Type 2 Diabetes Mellitus: A Double Blind Placebo Controlled Study," *Journal of the Association of Physicians of India* 49 (2001): 1057–1061.
80. Kouzi et al., "Natural Supplements for Improving Insulin Sensitivity and Glucose Uptake in Skeletal Muscle," 115.
81. The World's Healthiest Foods, "Clove," http://www.whfoods.com/genpage.php?tname=foodspiceanddbid=69.
82. R.P. Dearlove, "Inhibition of Protein Glycation by Extracts of Culinary Herbs and Spices," *Journal of Medicinal Food* 11(2) (2008): 275–281.
83. Shan et al., "Antioxidant Capacity of 26 Spice Extracts and Characterization of Their Phenolic Constituents," 7749.
84. S.S. Percival et al., "Bioavailability of Herbs and Spices in Humans as Determined by Ex Vivo Inflammatory Suppression and DNA Strand Breaks," *Journal of the American College of Nutrition* 31(4) (2012): 288–294.

85. H.A. Elwakeel, "Clove Oil Cream: A New Effective Treatment for Chronic Anal Fissure," *Colorectal Disease* 9(6) (2007): 549–552.

86. K. Pramod et al., "Eugenol: A Natural Compound with Versatile Pharmacological Actions," *Natural Product Communications* 5(12) (2010): 1999–2006.

87. H. Mith et al., "Antimicrobial Activities of Commercial Essential Oils and Their Components against Food-borne Pathogens and Food Spoilage Bacteria," *Food Science and Nutrition* 2(4) (2014): 403–416.

88. E. Darvishi et al., "The Antifungal Eugenol Perturbs Dual Aromatic and Branched-chain Amino Acid Permeases in the Cytoplasmic Membrane of Yeast," *PLoS ONE* 8(10) (2013): e76028.

89. The World's Healthiest Foods, "Fennel," http://www.whfoods.com/genpage.php?tname=foodspiceanddbid=23.

90. Münir Oktay et al., "Determination of In Vitro Antioxidant Activity of Fennel (*Foeniculum Vulgare*) Seed Extracts," *LWT-Food Science and Technology* 36(2) (2003): 263–271.

91. I. Alexandrovich et al., "The Effect of Fennel (Foeniculum Vulgare) Seed Oil Emulsion in Infantile Colic: A Randomized, Placebo-controlled Study," *Alternative Therapies in Health and Medicine* 9(4) (2003): 58–61.

92. V. Modaress Nejad and M. Asadipour, "Comparison of the Effectiveness of Fennel and Mefenamic Acid on Pain Intensity in Dysmenorrhoea," *Eastern Mediterranean Health Journal* 12(3–4) (2006): 423–427.

93. B. Singh and R.K. Kale, "Chemomodulatory Action of Foeniculum Vulgare (Fennel) on Skin and Forestomach Papillomagenesis, Enzymes Associated with Xenobiotic Metabolism and Antioxidant Status in Murine Model System," *Food and Chemical Toxicology* 46(12) (2008): 3842–3850.

94. Sarah Garland, *The Complete Book of Herbs and Spices* (New York: Reader's Digest, 1993), 48–50.

95. S. Sreelatha and R. Inbavalli, "Antioxidant, Antihyperglycemic, and Antihyperlipidemic Effects of Coriandrum Sativum Leaf and Stem in Alloxan-induced Diabetic Rats," *Journal of Food Science* 77(7) (2012): T119–123.

96. G. Park et al., "Coriandrum Sativum L. Protects Human Keratinocytes from Oxidative Stress by Regulating Oxidative Defense Systems," *Skin Pharmacology and Physiology* 25(2) (2012): 93–99.

97. R. Vejdani et al., "The Efficacy of an Herbal Medicine, Carmint, on the Relief of Abdominal Pain and Bloating in Patients with Irritable Bowel Syndrome: A Pilot Study," *Digestive Diseases and Sciences* 51(8) (2006): 1501–1507.
98. Aggarwal with Yost, *Healing Spices,* 103.
99. K. Srinivasan, "Plant Foods in the Management of Diabetes Mellitus: Spices as Beneficial Antidiabetic Food Adjuncts," *International Journal of Food Sciences and Nutrition* 56(6) (2005).
100. Sreelatha and Inbavalli, "Antioxidant, Antihyperglycemic, and Antihyperlipidemic Effects of Coriandrum Sativum Leaf and Stem in Alloxan-induced Diabetic Rats," 119–121.
101. P. Dhanapakiam et al., "The Cholesterol Lowering Property of Coriander Seeds (Coriandrum Sativum): Mechanism of Action," *Journal of Environmental Biology* 29(1) (2008): 53–56.
102. F. Casetti et al., "Antimicrobial Activity against Bacteria with Dermatological Relevance and Skin Tolerance of the Essential Oil from Coriandrum *Sativum* L. Fruits," *Phytotherapy Research* 26(3) (2012): 420–424.
103. F.C. Beikert et al., "Topical Treatment of Tinea Pedis Using 6% Coriander Oil in Unguentum Leniens: A Randomized, Controlled, Comparative Pilot Study," *Dermatology* 226(1) (2013): 47–51.
104. D.W. Unkle et al., "Anaphylaxis Following Cilantro Ingestion," *Annals of Allergy, Asthma and Immunology* 109(6) (2012): 471–472.
105. S. Sathyanarayana et al., "Unexpected Results in a Randomized Dietary Trial to Reduce Phthalate and Bisphenol A Exposures," *Journal of Exposure Science and Environmental Epidemiology* 23(4) (2013): 378–384.
106. L. Zhang and B.L. Lokeshwar, "Medicinal Properties of the Jamaican Pepper Plant Pimenta Dioica and Allspice," *Current Drug Targets*, December 2012, 13(14): 1900–1906.
107. Aggarwal with Yost, *Healing Spices*, 18–19.
108. R.P. Dearlove, "Inhibition of Protein Glycation by Extracts of Culinary Herbs and Spices," *Journal of Medicinal Food* 11(2) (2008): 275–281.
109. B.J. Doyle et al., "Estrogenic Effects of Herbal Medicines from Costa Rica Used for the Management of Menopausal Symptoms," *Menopause* 16(4) (2009): 748–755.
110. N. Shamaladevi et al., "Ericifolin: A Novel Antitumor Compound from Allspice that Silences Androgen Receptor in Prostate Cancer," *Carcinogenesis* 34(8) (2013): 1822–1832.
111. Aggarwal with Yost, *Healing Spices*, 19.

112. Garland, *The Complete Book of Herbs and Spices*, 90.

113. G. Kaur et al., "Modifying Anti-inflammatory Effect of Diclofenac with Murraya Koenigii," *Recent Patents on Inflammation and Allergy Drug Discoveries* 8(1) (2014): 77–81.

114. K. Srinivasan, "Plant Foods in the Management of Diabetes Mellitus: Spices as Beneficial Antidiabetic Food Adjuncts," *International Journal of Food Sciences and Nutrition* 56(6) (2005).

115. H. Yankuzo et al., "Beneficial Effect of the Leaves of Murraya Koenigii (Linn.) Spreng (Rutaceae) on Diabetes-induced Renal Damage In Vivo," *Journal of Ethnopharmacology* 135(1) (2011): 88–94.

116. Kaur et al., "Modifying Anti-inflammatory Effect of Diclofenac with Murraya Koenigii," 77–81.

117. M. Vasudevan and M. Parle, "Antiamnesic Potential of Murraya Koenigii Leaves," *Phytotherapy Research* 23(3) (2009): 308–316.

118. B. Noolu et al., "Murraya Koenigii Leaf Extract Inhibits Proteasome Activity and Induces Cell Death in Breast Cancer Cells," *BMC Complementary and Alternative Medicine* 13 (2013): 7.

119. Aggarwal with Yost, *Healing Spices*, 112.

120. M.H. Boskabady et al., "Carum Copticum L.: An Herbal Medicine with Various Pharmacological Effects," *BioMed Research International* 2014 (2014): 569087.

121. M.H. Boskabady, "Bronchodilatory Effect of Carum Copticum in Airways of Asthmatic Patients," *Therapie* 62(1) (2007): 23–29.

122. M.H. Boskabady et al., "Antitussive Effect of Carum Copticum in Guinea Pigs," *Journal of Ethnopharmacology* 97(1) (2005): 79–82.

123. K. Aftab et al., "Blood Pressure Lowering Action of Active Principle from Trachyspermum Ammi (L.) Sprague," *Phytomedicine* 2(1) (1995): 35–40.

124. A.H. Gilani et al., "Studies on the Antihypertensive, Antispasmodic, Bronchodilator and Hepatoprotective Activities of the Carumcopticum Seed Extract," *Journal of Ethnopharmacology* 98(1–2) (2005): 127–135.

125. Boskabady et al., "Carum Copticum L.: An Herbal Medicine with Various Pharmacological Effects," 569087.

126. J.A. Hawrelak et al., "Essential Oils in the Treatment of Intestinal Dysbiosis: A Preliminary In Vitro Study," *Alternative Medicine Review* 14(4) (2009): 380–384.

127. H.R. Sadeghnia et al., "Protective Effect of Safranal, a Constituent of Crocus Sativus, on Quinolinic Acid-induced Oxidative Damage in Rat Hippocampus," *Iranian Journal of Basic Medical Sciences* 16(1) (2013): 73–82.

128. Heather Ann Hausenblas et al., "Saffron (Crocus Sativus L.) and Major Depressive Disorder: A Meta-analysis of Randomized Clinical Trials," *Journal of Integrative Medicine* 11(6) (2013): 377–383.

129. S. Akhondzadeh et al., "A 22-Week, Multicenter, Randomized, Double-blind Controlled Trial of Crocus Sativus in the Treatment of Mild-to-moderate Alzheimer's Disease," *Psychopharmacology* (Berlin) 207(4) (2010): 637–643.

130. Sadeghnia et al., "Protective Effect of Safranal, a Constituent of Crocus Sativus, on Quinolinic Acid-induced Oxidative Damage in Rat Hippocampus," 73.

131. M. Agha-Hosseini et al., "Crocus Sativus L. (Saffron) in the Treatment of Pre-menstrual Syndrome: A Double-blind, Randomised and Placebo-controlled Trial," *BJOG: An International Journal of Obstetrics and Gynaecology* 115(4) (2008): 515–519.

132. Mohammad Heidary et al., "Effect of Saffron on Semen Parameters of Infertile Men," *Urology Journal* 5(4) (2008): 255–259.

**Chapter 8**

1. David Frawley, *Yoga and Ayurveda* (Silver Lake, WI: Lotus Press, 1999), 203–204.

2. Loren Cordain, *The Paleo Answer: 7 Days to Lose Weight, Feel Great, Stay Young* (Hoboken, NJ: John Wiley and Sons, 2012), 26–27.

3. Emily J. Dhurandhar et al., "The Effectiveness of Breakfast Recommendations on Weight Loss: A Randomized Controlled Trial," *American Journal of Clinical Nutrition* 100(2) (2014): 507–513.

4. Martin Berkhan, "The Leangains Guide," http://www.leangains.com/2010/04/leangains-guide.html.

5. Michael Mosley and Mimi Spencer, *The Fast Diet* (New York: Simon and Schuster, 2013).

6. James Johnson, "How to Do the Diet," http://www.johnsonupdaydowndaydiet.com/html/how-to-do-the-diet.html.

7. Ori Hofmekler, *The Warrior Diet* (Berkeley, CA: Blue Snake Books, 2007).

8. Brad Pilon, "Eat Stop Eat." http://www.eatstopeat.com/IFdiet.html.

9. Mosley and Spencer, *The Fast Diet,* 41–47.

**Chapter 9**

1. Kelly A. Shaw et al., "Exercise for Overweight or Obesity (Review)" *Cochrane Database of Systematic Reviews* (4) (2006), Art No. CD003817.
2. E.G. Trapp et al., "The Effects of High-intensity Intermittent Exercise Training on Fat Loss and Fasting Insulin Levels of Young Women," *International Journal of Obesity* (2008) 32, 684–691.
3. Department of the Army, *U.S. Army Fitness Training Handbook* (Guilford,CT: Lyons Press, 2003), 42.
4. M. Roig et al., "The Effects of Eccentric Versus Concentric Resistance Training on Muscle Strength and Mass in Healthy Adults: A Systematic Review with Meta-analysis," *British Journal of Sports Medicine* 43(8) (2009): 556–568.
5. Mathias Wernbom et al., "The Influence of Frequency, Intensity, Volume and Mode of Strength Training on Whole Muscle Cross-sectional Area in Humans," *Sports Medicine* 37(3) (2007): 225–264.
6. Jonathan Bailor, *The Calorie Myth: How to Eat More, Exercise Less, Lose Weight, and Look Better* (New York: HarperCollins, 2014), 241–259.
7. Doug McGuff and John Little, *Body by Science: A Research-based Program for Strength Training, Bodybuilding, and Complete Fitness in 12 Minutes a Week* (New York: McGraw-Hill, 2009).
8. Hidde P. van der Ploeg et al., "Sitting Time and All-cause Mortality Risk in 222,497 Australian Adults," *Archives of Internal Medicine* 172(6) (2012): 494–500.
9. Joan Vernikos, *Sitting Kills, Moving Heals* (Fresno, CA: Linden Publishing, 2011).
10. "Cardio or Weights: Which Comes First?," *Air Force News*, http://www.military.com/military-fitness/running/cardio-or-weights-which-comes-first.

**Chapter 10**

1. Centers for Disease Control and Prevention, "Insufficient Sleep Is a Public Health Epidemic," January 13, 2014 http://www.cdc.gov/features/dssleep/.
2. J.J. Gooley et al. "Exposure to Room Light before Bedtime Suppresses Melatonin Onset and Shortens Melatonin Duration in Humans," *Journal of Clinical Endocrinology and Metabolism* 96(3) (2011): E463–E472.
3. J.J. Gooley et al. "Exposure to Room Light before Bedtime Suppresses Melatonin Onset and Shortens Melatonin Duration in Humans," E463–E472.
4. M. Garaulet et al., "Timing of Food Intake Predicts Weight Loss Effectiveness," *International Journal of Obesity* 37 (2013): 604–611.

5. Jaminet and Jaminet, *Perfect Health Diet*, 376.
6. S.M. Schmid, "A Single Night of Sleep Deprivation Increases Ghrelin Levels and Feelings of Hunger in Normal-weight Healthy Men," *Journal of Sleep Research* 17 (2008): 331–334.
7. Arlet V. Nedeltcheva et al. "Insufficient Sleep Undermines Dietary Efforts to Reduce Adiposity," *Annals of Internal Medicine* 153(7) (2010): 435–441.
8. P.L. Turner and M.A. Mainster, "Circadian Photoreception: Ageing and the Eye's Important Role in Systemic Health," *British Journal of Opththalmology* 92(11) (2008):1439–1444.
9. C. Woodyard, "Exploring the Therapeutic Effects of Yoga and Its Ability to Increase Quality of Life," *International Journal of Yoga* 4(2) (2011):49–54.
10. N.K. Manjunath and S. Telles, "Influence of Yoga and Ayurveda on Self-rated Sleep in a Geriatric Population," *Indian Journal of Medical Research* 121 (2005): 683–690.
11. Lorenzo Cohen et al. "Psychological Adjustment and Sleep Quality in a Randomized Trial of Effects of a Tibetan Yoga Intervention in Patients with Lymphoma," *Cancer* 100(10) (2004): 2253–2260.
12. Kasiganesan Harinath et al. "Effects of Hatha Yoga and Omkar Meditation on Cardiorespiratory Performance, Psychologic Profile, and Melatonin Secretion," *Journal of Alternative and Complementary Medicine* 10(2) (2004): 261–268.
13. Carolyn Stoller et al. "Effects of Sensory-enhanced Yoga on Symptoms of Combat Stress in Deployed Military Personnel," *American Journal of Occupational Therapy*, 66 (2012): 59–68.
14. Woodyard, "Exploring the Therapeutic Effects of Yoga and Its Ability to Increase Quality of Life," 52–54.

**Chapter 11**

1. Hölzel BK et al., "Mindfulness Practice Leads to Increases in Regional Brain Gray Matter Density," *Psychiatry Research* 191(1) (2011): 36-43.
2. Hitendra Wadhwa, "Steve Jobs's Secret to Greatness: Yogananda," *Inc. Magazine*, June 21, 2015, http://www.inc.com/hitendra-wadhwa/steve-jobs-self-realization-yogananda.html.
3. Paramahansa Yogananda, *Spiritual Diary: An Inspirational Thought for Each Day of the Year* (Los Angeles: Self-Realization Fellowship, 1982), "July 13."
4. H.N. Rasmussen et al., "Optimism and Physical Health: A Meta-analytic Review," *Annals of Behavioral Medicine* 37(3) (2009): 239–256.

5. Harvard Medical School, "In Praise of Gratitude," *Harvard Mental Health Letter*, November 1, 2011, http://www.health.harvard.edu/newsletter_article/in-praise-of-gratitude.
6. L. Y. Thompson et al., "Dispositional forgiveness of self, others, and situations," *Journal of Personality*, 73(2) (2005): 313-59.
7. Alberto J. Espay et al., "Placebo Effect of Medication Cost in Parkinson Disease: A Randomized Double-blind Study," *Neurology* 84(8) (2015): 794–802.
8. Jay C. Fournier, et al., "Antidepressant Drug Effects and Depression Severity: A Patient-level Meta-analysis," *JAMA: Journal of the American Medical Association* 303(1) (2010): 47–53.
9. J.B. Moseley et al., "A Controlled Trial of Arthroscopic Surgery for Osteoarthritis of the Knee," *New England Journal of Medicine* 347(2) (2002): 81–88.
10. T.J. Kaptchuk et al., "Placebos Without Deception: A Randomized Controlled Trial in Irritable Bowel Syndrome," *PLoS ONE* 5(12) (2010): e15591.
11. C.A. Mouch and A.J. Sonnega, "Spirituality and Recovery from Cardiac Surgery: A Review," *Journal of Religion and Health* 51(4) (2012):1042–1060.
12. James Altucher, "10 Things I Learned from Richard Branson," February 2015, http://www.jamesaltucher.com/2015/02/10-things-i-learn-from-richard-branson/.

**Chapter 12**

1. N.M. Grindler, "Persistent Organic Pollutants and Early Menopause in US Women," *PLoS ONE* 10(1) (2015): e0116057.
2. Endocrine Society, "Endocrine Disrupting Chemicals," http://press.endocrine.org/edc.
3. S. Bae and Y.C. Hong, "Exposure to Bisphenol A from Drinking Canned Beverages Increases Blood Pressure: Randomized Crossover Trial," *Hypertension* 65(2) (2015):313–319.
4. Kristin Schafer et al., "Chemical Trespass: Pesticides in Our Bodies and Corporate Accountability," Pesticide Action Network North America, May 2004. http://www.panna.org/sites/default/files/ChemTresMain(screen).pdf.
5. Z. Walaszek et al., "Metabolism, Uptake, and Excretion of a D-Glucaric Acid Salt and Its Potential Use in Cancer Prevention," *Cancer Detection and Prevention* 21(2) (1997): 178–190.
6. Adams, *Probiotics: Protection Against Infection,* 231–234.

7. S.S. El-Kamary et al., "A Randomized Controlled Trial to Assess the Safety and Efficacy of Silymarin on Symptoms, Signs and Biomarkers of Acute Hepatitis," *Phytomedicine* 16(5) (2009): 391–400.

8. Nakazawa, *The Autoimmune Epidemic.*

9. Kelley Herring, "The Hidden Danger in Your Slow Cooker," February 26, 2014, http://blog.grasslandbeef.com/bid/89368/The-Hidden-Danger-in-Your-Slow-Cooker.

10. Environmental Working Group, "EWG's 2014 Shopper's Guide to Pesticides in Produce," http://www.ewg.org/release/ewgs-2014-shoppers-guide-pesticides-produce.

11. Environmental Working Group, "EWG's 2015 Shopper's Guide to Pesticides in Produce," http://www.ewg.org/foodnews/summary.php.

12. Schafer et al., "Chemical Trespass," Pesticide Action Network North America, May 2004. http://www.panna.org/sites/default/files/ChemTresMain(screen).pdf.

13. American Academy of Pediatrics, "Pesticide Exposure in Children," http://pediatrics.aappublications.org/content/130/6/e1765.full.pdf+html.

14. J.S. de Vendômois et al., "Debate on GMOs Health Risks after Statistical Findings in Regulatory Tests," *International Journal of Biological Sciences* 6(6) (2010): 590–598.

15. C. Gasnier et al., "Glyphosate-based Herbicides Are Toxic and Endocrine Disruptors in Human Cell Lines," *Toxicology* 262(3) (2009): 184–191.

16. A. Aris and S. Leblanc, "Maternal and Fetal Exposure to Pesticides Associated to Genetically Modified Foods in Eastern Townships of Quebec, Canada," *Reproductive Toxicology* 31(4) (2011): 528–533.

17. R. Mesnage et al. "Cytotoxicity on Human Cells of Cry1Ab and Cry1Ac Bt Insecticidal Toxins Alone or with a Glyphosate-based Herbicide," *Journal of Applied Toxicology*, 33 (2013): 695–699.

18. M. Gruzza et al., "Study of Gene Transfer In Vitro and in the Digestive Tract of Gnotobiotic Mice from Lactococcus Lactis Strains to Various Strains Belonging to Human Intestinal Flora," *Microbial Releases* 2(4) (1994): 183–189.

19. CCM, *Glyphosate China Monthly Report*, January 20, 2013, http://www.cnchemicals.com/PublishMaterial/860/Sample-Glyphosate%20China%20Monthly%20Report.pdf.

20. A. Samsel and S. Seneff, "Glyphosate, Pathways to Modern Diseases II: Celiac Sprue and Gluten Intolerance," *Interdisciplinary Toxicology* 6(4) (2013): 159–184.

21. Nathan Daley MD, "GMOs and Health: The Scientific Basis for Serious Concern and Immediate Action," June 9, 2013, http://www.greenmedinfo.com/blog/gmos-and-health-scientific-basis-serious-concern-and-immediate-action.
22. Anthony Samsel and Stephanie Seneff, "Glyphosate's Suppression of Cytochrome P450 Enzymes and Amino Acid Biosynthesis by the Gut Microbiome: Pathways to Modern Diseases," *Entropy* 15 (2013): 1416-1463.
23. Samsel and Seneff, "Glyphosate, Pathways to Modern Diseases II: Celiac Sprue and Gluten Intolerance," 159–184.
24. L. Hardell et al., "Exposure to Pesticides as Risk Factor for Non-Hodgkin's Lymphoma and Hairy Cell Leukemia: Pooled Analysis of Two Swedish Case-control Studies," *Leukemia and Lymphoma* 43(5) (2002): 1043–1049.
25. A.J. De Roos et al., "Cancer Incidence Among Glyphosate-Exposed Pesticide Applicators in the Agricultural Health Study," *Environmental Health Perspectives* 113(1) (2005): 49–54.
26. Kathryn Z. Guyton et al, "Carcinogenicity of Tetrachlorvinphos, Parathion, Malathion, Diazinon, and Glyphosate," *Lancet Oncology*, published online: March 20, 2015.
27. Gary M. Williams et al., "Safety Evaluation and Risk Assessment of the Herbicide Roundup and Its Active Ingredient, Glyphosate, for Humans," *Regulatory Toxicology and Pharmacology* 31(2) (2000), 117–165.
28. Juliette Legler et al., "Obesity, Diabetes and Associated Costs of Exposure to Endocrine Disrupting Chemicals in the European Union," *Journal of Clinical Endocrinology and Metabolism*, epub March 5, 2015.
29. US Centers for Disease Control and Prevention. Department of Health and Human Services, "Fourth National Report on Human Exposure to Environmental Chemicals" (2009), http://www.cdc.gov/exposurereport/pdf/FourthReport.pdf.
30. A.M. Calafat et al., "Exposure of the US Population to Bisphenol A and 4-Tertiary-Octylphenol: 2003–2004," *Environmental Health Perspectives* 116 (2008): 39–44.
31. Xiaoqian Gao et al., "Rapid Responses and Mechanism of Action for Low-dose Bisphenol S on*ex Vivo* Rat Hearts and Isolated Myocytes: Evidence of Female-specific Proarrhythmic Effects," *Environmental Health Perspectives*, Advance Publication: February 26, 2015, shttp://ehp.niehs.nih.gov/1408679/.
32. D.J. Watkins, "Exposure to PBDEs in the Office Environment: Evaluating the Relationships between Dust, Handwipes, and Serum," *Environmental Health Perspectives* 119 (9) (2011):1247–1252.

33. C.M. Butt, "Metabolites of Organophosphate Flame Retardants and 2-ethylhexyl Tetrabromobenzoate in Urine from Paired Mothers and Toddlers," *Environmental Science and Technology* 48(17) (2014):10432–10438.
34. T. Uchikawa et al., "Chlorella Suppresses Methylmercury Transfer to the Fetus in Pregnant Mice," *Journal of Toxicological Sciences* 36(5) (2011):675–680.

**Chapter 14**

1. S. Czernichow et al., "Effects of Long-Term Antioxidant Supplementation and Association of Serum Antioxidant Concentrations with Risk of Metabolic Syndrome in Adults," *American Journal of Clinical Nutrition* 90(2) (2009): 329–335.
2. Gerald Roliz, *The Pharmaceutical Myth: Letting Food Be Your Medicine Is the Answer for Perfect Health* (Pleasanton, CA: The Healing Body, 2012).
3. D.R. Davis et al., "Changes in USDA food composition data for 43 garden crops, 1950 to 1999," *Journal of the American College of Nutrition* 23(6) (2004):669–82.
4. F. Wolf and A. Hilewitz, "Hypomagnesaemia in Patients Hospitalised in Internal Medicine is Associated with Increased Mortality," *International Journal of Clinical Practice* 68(1) (2014): 111–116.
5. C. Coudray et al., "Study of Magnesium Bioavailability from Ten Organic and Inorganic Mg Salts in Mg-Depleted Rats Using a Stable Isotope Approach," *Magnesium Research* 18(4) (2005): 215–223.
6. Gruppo Italiano per lo Studio della Sopravvivenza nell'Infarto miocardico, "Dietary Supplementation with N-3 Polyunsaturated Fatty Acids and Vitamin E After Myocardial Infarction: Results of the GISSI-Prevenzione Trial," *Lancet* 354(9177) (1999): 447–455.

**Chapter 15**

1. Jaminet and Jaminet, *Perfect Health Diet*, 226–227.
2. Jaminet and Jaminet, *Perfect Health Diet*, 143–148.

# INDEX